D1564403

A DIET FOR 100 HEALTHY HAPPY YEARS

by Morvyth McQueen-Williams, M.D.
and Barbara Apisson
edited by Norman Ober

PRENTICE-HALL, INC., Englewood Cliffs, New Jersey

A DIET FOR 100 HEALTHY HAPPY YEARS
by Morvyth McQueen-Williams, M.D., and Barbara Apisson
edited by Norman Ober

Printed in the United States of America
Prentice-Hall International, Inc., London
Prentice-Hall of Australia, Pty. Ltd., Sydney
Prentice-Hall of Canada, Ltd., Toronto
Prentice-Hall of India Private Ltd., New Delhi
Prentice-Hall of Japan, Inc., Tokyo
Prentice-Hall of Southeast Asia Pte. Ltd., Singapore
Whitehall Books Limited, Wellington, New Zealand

10 9 8 7 6 5 4 3

Library of Congress Cataloging in Publication Data
McQueen-Williams, Morvyth.
A diet for 100 healthy, happy years.
Includes index.
1. Nutrition. 2. Longevity. 3. Centenarians–Caucasus. 4. Diet–Caucasus. 5. Reducing diets. 6. Cookery, Armenian. I. Apisson, Barbara, joint author. II. Title. [DNLM: 1. Diet–Popular works. 2. Nutrition–Popular works. WB400 M173d]
RA784.M3 1977 613.2 76–30710
ISBN 0–13–211185–3

Editor's Foreword

I met Dr. Morvyth McQueen-Williams in February 1974 at West Point Farms, Central Valley, New York. Barbara Apisson's food there has been enough to bring me up from Manhattan for over twenty-three years, but this time we had agreed to talk about writing a book. Barbara and Henri Apisson, the owners of this incomparable Orange County restaurant, warned in advance that I would find Dr. Williams brilliant and a challenge.

They were right on both counts. It has been a rewarding and often demanding relationship. We agreed up front that Dr. Williams would practice the medicine and that Barbara would assist with viewpoint, Caucasus data and the recipes you'll find in Chapters 10 and 11. Final language and format were my responsibility.

These barriers proved a little flexible. While Dr. Williams stoutly fought off my efforts to play doctor, the two women fenced with one another and with me over content, meaning and language. And I found Dr. Williams a relentless researcher with nearly total recall.

Morvyth labored during the week, assembling her data and typing up notes. When Barbara wasn't in the kitchen satisfying patrons, she scratched recipes on lined notepaper, consulted calorie charts, re-read books on the Caucasus, prodded her 92-year-old-mother's memory and prepared her defenses against our inevitable assaults. Midweek, the Apissons delivered fresh batches of Dr. Williams' notes to me in Manhattan. Weekends, I drove up with whatever I had typed for amplification, correction, polishing and debate. Sentiments at these sessions wavered between open hostility and mutual pleasure.

As the book reveals in detail, Dr. Williams was exposed repeatedly to radiation during her tenure at Johns Hopkins University and Hospital in Baltimore during the early 1940s. It is a singular testament to her brilliance and the validity of her work with her husband in botanicals that she fought off cancer's ravages for more than thirty years.

When our collaboration was in its second year, she began to lose her characteristic youthful and vigorous stance. Her imposing figure shrank to deepening sickness and, toward the end, infirmity. However, she suffered no loss in acuity of mind. Two weeks before she died on July 8, 1976, at Tuxedo Memorial Hospital, Tuxedo Park, New York, she told me she had fought cancer back for over thirty years and would do it again. As she said it, she clung to my hand with a show of affection and emotion I had not detected before.

There is something very revealing in her original Chapter 9 notes. I didn't know when I read them just how sick she was. During our sessions, she often talked about the need to present our facts ably enough to make readers believe the contents of the book. It was on her mind frequently. Toward autumn 1975 she wrote, "This book has just about gotten us off this planet. I feel the reader will sense the truth. In law, I understand that the dying man's testimony is given much credence. Facing eternity keeps a man from fabricating untruths." At the time, I thought she was being melodramatic even though I knew about what she called her "radiation sickness."

Before going on to her legacy to us, I think you should know something of the background of this exceptionally gifted woman.

Morvyth McQueen-Williams was descended from Swiss-born Jacques Necker, Louis XVI's controversial director general of finances and minister of state, and from his daughter, Germaine de Staël, an almost equally controversial literary and political salon mistress before the French revolutionary era.

Dr. Williams was identified early as one of Professor Lewis M. Terman's genius children (Terman-Binet, Stanford University). Professor Terman's final letter to the doctor states that no existing test standard was any longer able to measure her intelligence.

She received a B.A. at the University of California and with it the University Gold Medal as "the most distinguished student in the capacity of the University to reward."

After seven years of straight-A grades, Dr. Williams won her M.D. degree from Yale University, and later her M.A. and Ph.D. She was a certified medical specialist and served as a faculty member at Johns Hopkins University and Hospital, Baltimore, Maryland; and Institute of Pathology, Case Western Reserve, Cleveland, Ohio; Albany Medical College, Union University, Albany, New York; The University of California Medical School and Institute of Experimental Biology and Medicine; and Medical Center, now called Seton Hall University, South Orange, New Jersey.

The doctor's clinical notes and medical, biographical and medical news articles have been published widely. Dr. Williams was staff medical consultant to M.D. Publications, other medical educational organizations and Prentice-Hall. She held fellowships of the New Jersey Academy of Medicine, the American Academy of Geriatrics and the American Association for the Advancement of Science.

Dr. Williams was a Phi Beta Kappa. Her accomplishments led to life membership with the American Medical Writers Association, and membership in the International Academy of Preventive Medicine, American Medical Association, Johns Hopkins Medical and Surgical Association, Yale Medical Society, American Federation for Clinical Research and other organizations.

She married Kegan Sarkisian, a research phytologist and inventor in developmental physiology and nutritional sciences. Together they constructed a laboratory and completed patent work in methods of sex predetermination, means of enhancing germination and the propagation of seed plants, methods to control animal fertility, and other highly specialized projects in health, nutrition and survival.

This book is her effort to codify into a readable text more than twenty-five years of research and medical practice to help people live longer and better.

The food expert Dr. Williams has consulted and debated with in preparation of this book, Barbara Apisson, was born in Erzerum, Armenia, now part of Turkey. This mountainous Caucasus region, noted for the longevity of its inhabitants, kept its imprint on Barbara after she and her mother fled Turkey and settled in Massachusetts following World War I, keeping their traditions intact—and their recipes.

Barbara attended art school in Boston, and later studied design at Columbia University, New York City. She met Armenian-born Henri Apisson in New York in 1935. Henri's parents escaped with him to Marseilles, France, in the postwar period of Turkish extermination of Armenians. In 1930, graduating college in Berlin, he followed his three brothers, two sisters and parents to the United States, going into the furniture business in New York City.

Fulfilling a personal dream, the Apissons purchased the former Lewisohn estate in Central Valley, N. Y., in 1947. Both of the Apissons had, by then, been treated successfully by Dr. Max Gerson, lauded by John Gunther in the poignant book about his son's fatal illness, *Death Be Not Proud.* West Point Farms became a rarified retreat for Dr. Gerson's patients. For five years, Barbara supervised the kitchen, compared her own dietary theories with those of Dr. Gerson, and learned and built the skills that are the hallmark of the unique cuisine of the restaurant today.

Barbara also learned from visits with the famous Swiss clinician Dr. Max Bircher-Benner and the legendary Dr. Albert Schweitzer. She consulted both as she made better nutrition the goal of West Point Farms.

In her efforts for more than twenty-five years since the Gerson period, she has never been able to keep a chef. The soft-spoken, gentle Armenian lady with the silken silver-white hair brooks no compromise. And every chef exposed to her methods has concluded that she is bankruptcy-prone, a visionary spiking her creations with costly nutritive additives customers never know are there.

During the last two years of Dr. Williams' life, her companion, confidante and nurse was Barbara Apisson. This dedicated selfless lady has created a Shangri-la of her own. Deer and smaller animals roam unthreatened at West Point Farms. Dogs and cats, abandoned in the area, find their way there. One cat, Jolie, became a legend by surviving twenty-six years as a household pet.

The friendship of the Apissons and Sarkisians began in the early sixties. Word of the work of the doctor and her husband reached Barbara through a mutual friend familiar with Barbara's intense interest in nutrition. At first, the Apissons consulted Dr. Williams professionally.

The two women, Barbara and Morvyth, discovered how much they had in common. The extent of Dr. Williams' knowledge of and commitment to nutrition electrified Barbara. No medical person she had ever met before was so dedicated and aware. In addition, the two couples discovered that Henri and Kegan had spent their boyhoods within a few blocks of one another in Smyrna, Turkey, where their families had had businesses at the time.

Dr. Williams and her husband became habitués of West Point Farms. When the doctor saw Barbara's organic gardens for the first time and began to appreciate the West Point Farms commitment to nutritional cookery, it was inevitable that the two women should begin thinking about writing a book together, based on the food and health habits of the Caucasus after the Sarkisians' 1968 studies in the region.

Only a few intimates know the doctor's dogged struggle to see this book through and Barbara Apisson's efforts to give Dr. Williams some of her own strength as the doctor's failed. One of those intimates was

Norman Ober

Contents

Introduction

We've always searched for a fountain of youth. Adventurers have scoured the earth hunting for something that lies within each of us, available for use. When nourished right and working properly, our bodies *are* fountains of youth, maintaining and regenerating us. When nourished and managed badly, our bodies go awry, we get sick often and we die prematurely.

My years of practicing medicine have convinced me that the benefits of civilization and technology have unintentionally but inevitably weaned us from the survival and health practices our ancestors relied on when survival was a full-time necessity. As science and medicine have registered awesome gains on the killers and on the life span itself, natural protective methods and survival folklore have fallen into disuse. Humankind has become overconfident, over-reliant on technology, and has forgotten history. If we would simply utilize our modern gains without abandoning what the past has taught us about survival, wouldn't we be far better off as a species?

My exposure to the role of nutrition in health and longevity began when, as a teen-ager, I was fortunate enough to become part of the research team of Dr. Herbert McLean Evans at the University of California. I was on my way to becoming a doctor, already totally fascinated with the potential and magnificence of the human body.

Dr. Evans and his senior staff, dedicated nutritional scientists, scored significant advances through their studies of known human ailments in animals. Their goal was to find out why our bodies go wrong when they do and how to remedy, or better still, prevent the ailments. Dr. Evans felt his work could create nutritional standards that would rescue millions from a growing list of illnesses directly or indirectly related to defective diets.

At Berkeley, we examined the overall effects of one illness after another caused by diet deficiency. For each set of sick animals, we fanatically maintained carefully fed controls of the same species. We observed and recorded the manifestations of the sick. At the same time, we observed and recorded the behavior of the healthy. Painstakingly, we proved not only that dietary differences were making one group healthy and the other sick, but precisely what deficiencies caused the illnesses.

There was no known deficiency I didn't work on personally during six rewarding years with Dr. Evans and his hematologists, chemists, clinicians, biochemists, physiologists, nutritionists and endocrinologists, so motivated, precise and selfless.

Soon I designed my own experiments; made up feeds, dietary and hormonal preparations and extracts; and fed rats by the thousands, as well as mice, guinea pigs and rabbits. I recorded results daily, compiled scientific observations, conducted examinations of animal organs and tested tissues for evidence and effects of abnormalities.

I recorded appearances of brown muscles; diseased hearts; palsied, dragging limbs in animals lacking just one nutrient, first known in our laboratory as vitamin X, later named vitamin E. With vitamins A, B, C and D identified by then, the next available letter was E, but I like to think of it as E for Evans, who discovered it.

Widely accepted for some human needs today, vitamin E is still under intense study by clinicians and nutritionists and considered controversial when promoted as a defense against heart and blood-vessel disorders. But even if we can't yet fully explain it, none of us who were at Berkeley with Dr. Evans doubts the great value of vitamin E in heart and blood-vessel diseases, in disorders of the muscles and sex organs, and in other problems brought on by vitamin-E deficiency and then cured by its addition to the diet.

Our research didn't stop there. We studied rats on low-protein diets; rats on caloric restraint; rats deficient in vitamin A, the various B vitamins and vitamin D; rats lacking unsaturated fats; rats with every dietary abnormality we could think of. We found out what happens to bodies deprived of nutrients through ignorance, fads or the bad eating habits to which people are subject.

Through these studies we learned how to prevent, with improved nutrition, dwarfism, skin disturbances, vision impairments, abnormal overgrowth, neurological problems, diabetes, kidney malfunction, pituitary imbalance, sex-function loss and many other disabilities. The only difference between what kept our animals healthy and what made them sick was the food they ate.

Animals damaged by poor diet faded, suffered and, if unaided, died prematurely. Those on balanced diets enjoyed full, normal lives for their species. Understanding these documented research findings at Berkeley will prepare you to stop attacking *your* fountain of youth through deficient diet, to power it up for extra years through proper nutrition. What's in our regimen for you? For your children? A fuller life span for you, an even fuller one for them.

Is it possible that you and I can be somehow different from people more than half a world away who live not just to the age of 100, but to 130, 140, 150 and beyond? I propose to you now that if their oldest recorded life span is 178, with an average of 62 more per 100,000 of them living past the century mark than us, there *is* something different about them, about their bodies, their durability. But if you have the will and motivation to work along with us on the regimen detailed and explained in this book, then we have a package of living habits, nutrients, supplements, exercises, ways of preparing food and foods to avoid—a way to live better and longer that depends on *you*. *You* learning, *you* doing. *You* counting on *you*. Interested?

1.

Self-Pollution Made Easy

The job of fortifying the young begins before conception. I hope to persuade you that optimum health and maximum longevity demand a lifetime of proper attention to nutrition. Proper attention to diet before and during the childbearing years produces healthy children. For your own health and for longer life, please consider proper nutrition a lifetime concern with few, if any, times out.

Merely cutting back on indulgences is not the answer. Sporadic binges of well-intentioned starving, like binges of uncontrolled eating, are likely to eliminate necessary vitamins, minerals, vegetable oils, fruits and vegetables.

Did you begin your breakfast with frozen orange juice this morning? You might have read on the container, if you bothered, that there is citric acid in what you are drinking.

Perhaps after your juice, because you like to watch your weight, you ate packaged cereal with powdered nonfat dry milk dissolved in water. Listed among other ingredients on the cereal box is "BHT added" or its equivalent. Or maybe you had bacon and eggs this morning. The bacon package says sodium phosphate, sodium erythorbate and sodium nitrite have been added. They are not nutrients. They give artificial color to the meat.

If you had toast, the bread wrapper probably said sodium propionate or its like has been added to preserve freshness. Did you use margarine on the toast? The container says the product contains partially hydrogenated corn oil, vegetable mono- and diglycerides, potassium sorbate and calcium disodium EDTA as preservatives.

And very likely you had coffee with its caffeine.

That's breakfast for millions, give or take a few or many of these or other chemicals that I call pollutants deliberately and voluntarily ingested.

So to lunch. Sandwich with mayonnaise? Mayonnaise means more EDTA (ethylinediaminetetraacetic acid) inside of you. Coffee or cola? More caffeine. And in the cola is some unidentified substance called "artificial coloring." If you had a carbonated diet drink to spare your waistline, most likely it contained sodium gluconate, citric acid, saccharin, sodium citrate, artificial coloring and sodium benzoate—a chemical cocktail. The bread in your sandwich (like your morning toast) provides more sodium propionate, chemical coloring, hydrogenated fat and many many more additives. Bread can contain sixty additives many of which are not required to be on the label. An example is calcium bromate, a dough ripener, not listed because the law doesn't insist that small amounts of chemicals used in processing be shown on the label. Bread may have some sixteen chemicals in it just to keep it fresh. The label doesn't list them all or even most of them.

Ready for dinner? You might begin with a minced clam appetizer, sodium triphosphate added. Use chili and horseradish from a bottle and you're apt to find on the label the "harmless" information that dehydrated onion and "flavoring" have been added, with no hint of what the flavoring is nor of what dehydration has cost the onions in food value.

Green salad with prepared dressing? The salad-dressing bottle advertises "modified food starch added." That isn't too reassuring if you know anything about modifying processes. Then there's that unexplained ingredient "flavor" again and more calcium disodium EDTA to protect that flavor.

Let's say your main course is a packaged convenience food. In it, your day's additives spurt ahead with dehydrated beef, undefined starch, dehydrated vegetables (more original food values processed out), hydrogenated vegetable oils, vegetable gums, hydrolized plant protein, monosodium glutamate, flavorings, colorings, tricalcium phosphate and BHA added as an antioxidant. All of the above is off one label for a beef and noodle product.

If you stick to fresh meat and vegetables, you still run into additives that are put in to retard spoilage, improve color, improve texture, and so on.

Let's add as dessert a modest commercial gelatin product. That supplies you with more hydrogenated vegetable oil, sugar, adipic acid, polyglycerol esters of fatty acids, artificial flavor and color and more BHA.

Olives from a bottle because you like them? Ferrous gluconate added. Pickles? Polysorbate 80 added. And over and over again in these foods we see sugar added, salt added, without any way whatever of finding out how much of any of these ingredients get into us each time we eat. And if you chance to switch to a low-calorie sugar substitute for "health reasons," the cure may be worse than the disease because of saccharin, calcium chloride and artificial flavor and color, undefined, added.

Move in any direction you like from the sample meal I've put together above and you will total up, day after day, a staggering number of additives accomplishing various commercial purposes but having little or nothing to do with nutrition.

They are not necessarily all bad but many have acquired bad reputations in laboratory work you know little or nothing about. The appearance of any of these additives on the official Food and Drug Administration (FDA) GRAS (Generally Recognized as Safe) list isn't too reassuring. I can't tell you that the record of the FDA is good in outlawing suspect additives. It takes a great deal to make the FDA suspicious. There is a discouraging number of cases in which evidence that an additive is unsafe is heeded in other countries but not here.

There is ample documented reading available to you if you want to learn more about this painful subject. The point I want to make now is that neither you, nor I, nor the FDA, nor the food industry has the foggiest notion of what all those allowed additives, numbering some 4,000 by this date, *in combination,* are doing to our bodies. No team of scientists can recreate in a laboratory the cumulative effects of all the pollutants we eat in our food day after day.

Nutritionists worry about synergistic effect. In our context, synergistic means that, while one chemical alone may show no harmful effects when taken into the body, for reasons not always clear, the same chemical taken with some other chemical, possibly also harmless when taken by itself, can, in combination, turn out to be harmful or even fatal.

By some standard, often questionable, each additive is tested and an amount allowed which is presumably not harmful to you. But nobody can measure the toxicity potentials of all those combinations of additives pouring into us daily, or to what extent synergistic effect may be piling up to create, in short term or over the years, heart disease, cancer and other killers.

It is not my design to analyze, chemical by chemical, what is wrong with all those additives I mentioned in my sample meal. If you want, your librarian can make available to you books that delve deeply into this subject. Be sure you ask for scientific and authoritative texts, not faddish and sensational treatments. The sober facts are bad enough.

You will learn how much is already known about many of these additives that preserve freshness and color in our food, and particularly about experiments that show danger of cancer and other unlooked-for results from all this chemistry. You may then understand why more and more people, alarmed as I am alarmed, are turning away from processed foods to natural foods.

We have had far too few Herbert McLean Evanses leading the way within organized medicine. Only lately are we observing within medicine and on the parts of individual doctors interest in food as curative and preventive medicine. At least partly, that's why we are, as a nation, in deep trouble with our diets, running out of advantages from scientific gains, losing ground.

I am convinced that the medical profession must take and keep the initiative in nutritive health. The public is entitled to this interest and service from us.

While we are learning more about nutrition all the time, it is a great temptation to doctors to concentrate on healing the sick, a large enough task in our society, and to ignore the far better course of preventive medicine. As a way of starting, I cordially invite my fellow doctors, for their own health as well as for their patients', to become better informed on the terrifying role of additives in commercial food.

Additives are only part of the story. I tell my patients, "Don't buy nonfat dry milk powder." Here, the bigger problem is processing. Too often, processors (as of nonfat dry milk) are not required to put on the box what they have added. And the problem of *subtractives* is just as large.

Much of today's milk processing wastes nutritives, uses them up, destroys them. Skimming milk removes vitamins. Heat-drying it burns up food values. It will not surprise you that our regimen shuns processed food and emphasizes reliance on natural, unprocessed and minimally cooked foods. In places we'll tell you about, people have been enjoying better health, better sex and longer life on natural foods for centuries, without benefit of the latest wonders of science. It's time harried Americans "discovered" those foods.

Processing turns brown sugar into white, unbleached flour into white. White flour and white sugar are two major villains on our nutrient scene. With the American dollar buying less, in the name of health and longer life, available food money should be channeled away from refined white sugar and refined white flour as the nutritionally deficient body fodder they are.

I've often talked about self-pollution to my patients. The 170 pounds of white sugar a year Americans pour into themselves is one of our chief self-pollutants. And think, we've been conditioned to do this to ourselves.

You can begin correcting this condition by baking your own bread. If you do, you'll be converting your family to a highly nutritious, chemical-free product far better for you than most of what's on your store's shelves today. There are two excellent bread recipes in Chapter 11 and more available in cookbooks for breads *you* bake, using soy, millet and other whole-grain products alone or in combinations. Look for them.

Massive home bread baking is the only way we're ever going to get our vast commercial baking companies to put nutrition ahead of shelf life and provide a staff of life that doesn't let us down over the long haul.

Yes, you *can* bake your own breads. You *can*, if you will, join growing legions who raise organically some of their own fruit and vegetables. We may not soon totally escape additives in our diets (nor even want to escape them all), but we can reduce our intakes of them sharply by careful buying. You can band together in shopping pools to buy direct from food wholesalers, saving money and cutting down on the time that elapses before food gets to your table.

I am convinced that, for many, your very life is at stake if you don't help yourself out of the trap by enlightenment and a change of your entire approach to eating such as you'll read about in later chapters.

Before I get into other matters, let me add that I am not keen on honey, brown sugar and maple sugar as substitutes for white sugar. Although less harmful than white sugar, they all contribute to polluting the body through excessive carbohydrate intake. Quit white sugar and use as little as possible of the others. Our diet and maintenance chapters will give you days of meals de-emphasizing, though not eliminating, trouble-maker carbohydrates. We do need some carbohydrates. Getting enough is no problem. They occur naturally in grains, fruit, vegetables and in protein-containing foods. Our American romance with sweets simply gives us vast quantities of carbohydrates above what we need and get naturally in good foods, overloading our systems and, in concert with excess calories, fatiguing our hearts, stunting energy production, creating gastrointestinal havoc, assaulting our vital sources and forces.

Self-pollution, as you can see, *is* easy. It has been made easy for us by food chemistry and food processing that affect a greater and greater proportion of our available food supply. You can reduce the effects of polluted food on your family by the way you buy and the way you prepare your family's food. You'll learn a great deal about how to do that as you continue to read.

2. Where Centenarians Love Life

My husband and I worked and studied in the Caucasus in 1968. Do you know where it is? Many Americans call themselves Caucasians and scarcely know why.

The Caucasus, or Transcaucasia, is in southeastern U.S.S.R. It extends from the Caucasus mountain range on the north and continues southward between the Black and Caspian seas. It is bounded by Turkey on the west and Iran on the south and southeast.

The ancient history of the area is one of fluid boundaries. Much of what was once Armenia is now eastern Turkey. People with roots in the region tend to think of that sector, as well as the land just north of the Caucasus mountains and adjacent parts of Iran and Iraq, as Caucasus country, with considerable ethnic evidence to support their claims. It is Garden of Eden and Mount Ararat land, where more than legend indicates that mankind established the first beachhead on earth somewhere in the area's favorable soil, vegetation, water and air expanse.

I contend to you, as I see humanity racing toward technologically accelerated doom, that the only hope left to us is to return figuratively to Edenland and to rediscover what centuries of surviving hardships taught our Caucasian ancestors. My husband, Kegan, and I embarked on our personal rediscovery route during three months of tests of our botanical method of attacking cancer. We were guests of the Soviet government. We treated and interviewed many patients and took advantage of the opportunity to test healthy as well as sick people, many of them elderly.

We queried oldsters who happened to be Georgian, Azerbaijani, Armenian, Nakhichevani, Daghestan, Abkhaz, Adzhar, Jew or transplanted Muscovite. We quickly discovered that the region's elderly have one thing in common: all are on natural diets, eating organic food fresh from their own soil, self-cultivated, additive-free, balanced in natural vitamins, minerals and whole grains, and avoiding processed white flour or white sugar.

Who kept these secrets alive? Who developed what Kegan and I discovered during three months of interviews, note taking, researching? Kegan had said it was the Armenians, the oldest surviving people of the region. Barbara Apisson *knew* it was the Armenians. Her mother said *everyone* knew it. Most everyone we asked who had an opinion seemed to agree, barring a certain amount of ethnic rivalry. We saw for ourselves that people in the Caucasus, living a century and longer, numbering as many as one-fourth of the populations of some villages we visited, were all eating by the centuries-old rules of their Armenian neighbors.

How did Armenians' methods survive since earlier than written records? Over seventy years ago, when Kegan and Henri Apisson were born in what is now Turkish Armenia, itinerant storytellers still visited the villages, staying here a week and there two, singing songs and repeating tales that had been told to them, to their parents and to their parents' parents.

Their songs were of bravery, of survival, of overcoming great odds. Among them were recitals of how to till the rich soil for optimum yields, how to plough, plant, grow, husband, harvest —even how to prepare and how to eat the region's natural abundance. These songs and recitals were repeated by generations of storytellers, the historians and naturalists of their time.

The health attributes of each food, each recipe, each combination of ingredients were thus conveyed and kept alive to benefit those who understood what it had taken to survive in primitive times.

Some 6,500 years ago, the Neolithic revolution took place in the area. Man revolted against feast or famine, against a diet of raw food that tortured and killed when eaten stale. He learned. He adapted. He tamed wild animals, cultivated plants, kept bees, built his home near the productive soil and mineral-rich water. He slowly abandoned the primitive ways of wide-range foraging for survival in favor of a personal planned economy. This spared his nerves and legs for a gradually lengthening life span. And his thoughts turned to what each generation since must have regarded as the better things in life.

The Armenians, despite frequent sweeping invasions, developed this way. They are the only surviving tribe whose ancestry began in Edenland. It is no shame learning from survival-wise teachers. When you consider how many concerted efforts there were to engulf them, overwhelm them or eradicate them, their endurance stands as one of history's great miracles.

Prey in turn to Mongolians, Babylonians, Persians, Arabs, Turks and others, marked for extermination again this same century, phoenix-like, they have survived and multiplied, always replacing their losses. Recorded as great fighters against fantastic odds, they survived not because of weaponry but because, all these years, they have known better how to nourish and strengthen their minds and bodies than have their attackers. Added to the Armenians' natural practices, today's health breakthroughs should see us all living well into our second centuries.

Is their history fantasy or is there proof that the early Armenians' grains were as nutritious as today? Did the original Caucasian really get ample vitamin C in his fruits? Did his fish, meat, vegetables, greens, seeds provide the rich protein, calcium, iron and minerals for strong bones and teeth, full vitamin values and the fifty-to-sixty-item nutrient string today known to shore up body, mind and sexuality?

Bones excavated in digs support such speculation. Studies of paintings, scrawls and carvings give evidence that large families were normal and attest to the strong sexual powers of these people. Seeds and grains buried for centuries and uncovered in searches show fine protein content, excellent unsaturated fat composition. Skull findings attest to good dental arch patterns and excellent teeth. Judging from bony markings, muscles must have been tremendous, exactly as sung generation after generation by the storytellers.

One of their proudest legends: David of Sassoon was consulted by the elders on how to rid the region of a man-eating lion. David knew his strength. He would dispose of the marauder on its next prowl for human flesh. As soon as the lion appeared, he loaded himself down with weapons and confronted the enemy. But when he saw the lion, David suddenly knew he must meet the great beast on equal terms. Each intent on survival, it was unfair to weigh the odds in David's favor with weapons.

David shed his weapons and stepped out to meet the lion with only his large bare hands and strong body. Could muscles, bone and brain overcome the brute ferocity of the animal? David won the battle and moved into Armenian history as a folk hero.

Many similar legends remain as symbols of a love of life that characterizes these people. It is evident, too, in the care with which they learned to sound their soils, plumb the waters, understand the vegetation and know nature well enough in sum to produce our Caucasus diet.

The Neolithic Caucasians gave up eating grubs, larvae and insects. They found that hunting, fishing, berrying, planting and cultivating unmilled natural grains were far better substitutes, strengthening them, enlarging their pelvic girdles, building great vertebrae and shoring up their skeletal systems.

From these early beginnings, the Caucasus way has continued to this day to enrich and strengthen its fortunate people in the favored region that opened its arms to receive Kegan and me in 1968.

I have telescoped centuries into pages for a purpose. You see, I didn't marry Kegan Sarkisian as a believer. And I didn't become one overnight. It took my research and medical practice, my growing experience in the science of nutrition, the role of nutrition in health and longevity, and exposure to the Caucasus elders themselves to make me believe in and work with the relationship between nutrition and longer, healthier years.

Caucasus health experts wanted to know more about our use of botanicals as health aids, discoveries we made based on Kegan's years of study and research that began in that part of the world.

Kegan attended Mechitarist College in Smyrna and, later, the American University in Constantinople as a foreign student. His studies there were interrupted by World War I.

Kegan came to the United States in 1919. He spent four years at the University of New Hampshire, specializing in genetic research in agriculture, studies he had begun in the schools of his homeland. As a boy, he had worked in a family business involving the manufacture and sale of medications from botanical sources. At the University of New Hampshire, he introduced beekeeping by the methods of his ancestors. In this period, he was also involved with development of the New Hampshire Red, a superior hen species.

I met Kegan in 1945 in Englewood, New Jersey, while I was still on staff at Johns Hopkins. I was on temporary leave during one of my early periods of radiation sickness, a product of doctors' own ignorance of the dangers of X-ray that has haunted me ever since my exposures in connection with my work at Hopkins. I'll talk about that later, since I must. During my leave, I was visiting a doctor friend in Englewood. He introduced me to Kegan. Two months later we were married.

Soon we formulated plans for a home and laboratory. We began our joint research in our apartment near Gracie Mansion in New York City while our home was being built in Englewood Cliffs.

Some very rewarding things happened in a short time. Before the end of World War II, we signed a contract with the U.S.

Army to develop a butter substitute. The Office of Price Administration pronounced it acceptable. As we moved toward production, the war ended. The Army lost interest. Kegan took it stoically. He spoke sparingly and softly with an Armenian accent. "Janeeg," he said, "we'll try again." Janeeg was his nickname for me.

In 1951, we moved to Englewood Cliffs. Our work in nutrition continued. Kegan had interests without end. A genetic system he invented was sold in 1954, netting $1 million for its buyers in three months.

In 1958, King Ranch of Texas purchased our process for sex predetermination for animals. We were on our way. I developed a medical practice. As time permitted, Kegan and I worked together in the lab. The early profitable work we did was involved in animal nutrition, but we were learning the power of vitamins and minerals found in natural herbs and botanicals.

We learned a great deal about the constituency of many fresh natural herbs and demonstrated their value as sources of supply superior to conventional food acquired in the conventional way. We soon demonstrated with living patients how damaged bodies responded to nutritional attack. Our work came to the attention of our counterparts in the Soviet Union, and we were invited there in 1968 under the sponsorship of the Chief Minister of Health of the U.S.S.R., Dr. Boris Petrovsky. He sent us to Yerevan (Erivan) University as official guests of the State.

Before I go into our observations and experiences on that trip, I should add a little more about Kegan. He suffered from the Kennedy syndrome, a variety of Addison's disease. The condition began in World War II when he injured his spine saving two girls from drowning. It eventually became stabilized. He learned to live with it and ignored his pains as much as he could, but in 1972 he accidentally wrenched his back, reinjured his spine and suffered a full return of symptoms. In early 1973, he was in such pain that we decided on hospital rest and treatment. He went to St. Michael's Hospital, Newark, New Jersey, where he died suddenly and unexpectedly of complications.

At the time of his death, Kegan was incumbent John F. Kennedy Award winner for excellence in medical research and service to the national community. My memory of this is reinforced by a Kennedy bust and citation.

To get back to our Caucasus travels in 1968, I had begun to tell you that, in effect, my late husband was, as I think back on it, bringing to their source his laboratory discoveries based on his family's generations of medicinal use of herbs and botanicals. We proved many of his family's theories in our laboratory, isolating the vitamins and minerals in concoctions his ancestors had invented in their time.

Kegan and I left the Caucasus with profound new appreciation for natural organic cultivation and dietary habits that brought a people back from near extinction to some eight million around the world today. Not surprisingly, the first time I visited Barbara Apisson's wonderful gardens at West Point Farms I saw the same organic methods producing prodigious quantities of fresh food.

Naturally, our studies in the Caucasus accelerated my interest in longevity. Longevity is everywhere there—old people erect and active in their eighties, nineties and beyond, up to a century and a half and more. It still sobers me to compare their centenarians, measured by the Armenian government at an average of 65 per 100,000, with the bare 3 per 100,000 we count in the United States.

In this connection, in the June 1976 issue of *Soviet Life,* which Barbara Apisson excitedly brought me, I read an article about longevity in the Caucasus that would have drawn cheers from Kegan. The author, Vladimir Kyucharyants, tells of finding oldsters in great numbers everywhere in the Caucasus. Then comes this line: "Honors go to Azerbaijan, more precisely the Nagorny Karabakh Region, where approximately 100 out of every 100,000 are over a century old." Kegan would have cheered because that area used to be part of Armenia. The figure thrilled me because it's the highest I have ever seen.

It's easy to scoff at what one hasn't seen. But like Kyucharyants, the author in *Soviet Life,* we found large populations of the elderly who were active, looking really alive. They worked in the fields, prepared the food and worked part-time, if not full-time. They were not aging vegetables cast aside by society. Instead, they had meaningful roles in urban life and in the more demanding existence of their highland villages.

The oldest ones we observed walked with spring in their steps, moved as though, if need be, they could leap to the attack. A common sight almost everywhere was an oldster trotting as though late, a basket of produce, fresh from the fields, in his arms.

I clapped my hands with pleasure when a copy of an Armenian paper (*Armenian Reporter,* January 3, 1974) front-paged a photo of a man named Gabriel Chapnian, describing him as "Indefatigable at age 117." In 1968, he was a hundred and eleven and introduced to us as Gabrielovich Chiapavelly. He was a showpiece of his local Abkhazian region of the Caucasus. The paper's caption quotes his prescription for longevity: "Active physical work and a moderate interest in alcohol and the ladies."

His being called Chiapavelly stemmed from Georgian pride. The Russians had us in charge. They Georgianized his name to Chiapavelly to convince us that he was really Russian. But Kegan wasn't taken in. He knew the man by his quizzical eyes and prominent brows, what Kegan called "almond eyes." A question in Armenian settled the issue, although the old gentleman acknowledged some Georgian blood, too.

When we met him, although a pensioner, he was working full-time. He wore his service pin over his heart. He had good eyesight, good hearing, powerful legs, arms and neck. Mentally, he was alert and bright.

Kegan asked Chapnian-Chiapavelly what luck had brought him to his advanced age. "Luck? We got rid of the enemy in 1917."

Kegan had a way of plumbing the old man's interest in sex. He asked a question in Armenian. The old man beamed. "Naturally, my boy, whenever I can get my hands on them." He was not bragging about women, at least not directly. He was confessing to a taste for what's referred to in nicer circles as lamb fry (pan-fried testicles of lamb), firmly believed to impart to partakers extra reserves of sexual prowess. See our recipes for it in Chapters 10 and 11.

This didn't surprise Kegan. Hadn't his cousin the Bear-Choker told Kegan that his great-uncle the Pony Express Rider also had partaken of this superfood? How else, it was understood, did that stalwart rise to the opportunities of his stopovers during the long overland gallops?

What did Chapnian eat when there were no lamb's testes to fry? The staples he enumerated we heard again and again, not just from Armenians in the area but from elderly Moslems there, Jews, and, as noted, all the diverse elderly peoples who populate the Caucasus.

We found the same basic diet in the highlands, along the Black Sea coast, bordering the Caspian, up in the rural plateaus and down in the cities. Kegan thought all the oldsters there would prove to be Armenian. Not so. But as scientists, we were excited to see a commonality of diet as one of the empirical dominants of our research.

Jew, Gentile, Moslem, every aging ethnic division we observed consumed more grain protein than meat protein. Meats were lean, the area's fish were lean. Nonsaturated vegetable fats were favored. A minimum of animal fat is used in the Caucasus. The people tended to live on yogurt, sour milks and homemade unfatty cheeses. Their carbohydrates came chiefly from homemade whole-grain breads. Their sweets were mostly fruits. They doted on green salads and, except in winter, ate a large variety of fresh-grown vegetables. In Chapter 8, when we describe Barbara Apisson's garden, you'll discover that proper care produces vegetables fresh from the ground even after the weather turns cold.

Kegan and I made notes on a good number of oldsters, not all of them by name. There was a ninety-year-old pensioner in Erivan, an ex-official who had worked in Moscow, Georgia and Armenia and who had retired the year we saw him. He enjoyed being questioned.

This charming gentleman, being only ninety, was in Erivan for two reasons. He was there for the ongoing celebration of "2750" and he was also, he confided, wife hunting. The observance of "2750" was held in 1968 by sixteen Soviet republics in honor of the discovery, through cuneiform markings, of proof of the age of a historic fort. It was considered a triumph for Armenia's claims to primacy in Western architectural forms.

Our ex-official acknowledged to Kegan that he, too, was a lamb-fry devotee, "Whenever and wherever I can get my hands on them." I think there is a good deal to the belief that lamb fries offer an extra bonus in sex. But true or not, if the world is ever made over in Armenia's image, lambs will grow dozens of testes.

This retired oldster told me, "My prospective wife will love our traditions. She will know how to prepare chick-peas with *tahini* for the added strength it will give me. And *tarama* [pink caviar]! And if she serves me *midia dolma* [stuffed mussels], a must for lovers, what more could I ask of her?"

We learned more than this man's favorite dishes for virility. As with Gabriel Chapnian, all the tried-and-true dishes from antiquity were on his list. He favored me with *sotto voce* explanations of just how each traditional dish came into being, all the way from earliest recorded history and legend to the origins of Armenia's pre-Christian monasteries. He was a treasure, that lively wife hunter.

Another delightful, highly intelligent oldster we met was Mrs. Kenleyan, Kegan's grandaunt. I snapped four generations of her family in one photo. She's an excellent multigrain bread baker, an avid reader and a magical hand with the fruit of *Prunus armeniaca* (apricots), grapes, *petmez*, *tahini* and almond paste, and conserve of green nuts served as sweets. Her staples mirrored what we found on tables throughout the region: eggplant, okra, squash, cucumber, herbs, botanicals (where needed), *bulgur* pilaf, fish, lamb, chicken and, for herself, a thimbleful of grape wine or Armenian cognac for toasts. All of the above was presented in one meal she served me with Kegan absent. She herself ate sparingly of what she provided to welcome the doctor from "Ameri*cahhh.*"

Mrs. Kenleyan, going strong at the age of 105, was given a helpful shot by a Westernized doctor, and her sight went suddenly dim. It severely restricted her reading, a great tragedy.

We also visited Mrs. Vorperian, discreet about her exact age but nearing 100, still conducting lavish outdoor kabobs. As the century mark neared, she gave up growing her own garden. But she made regular trips to a nearby park to enjoy the flowers and visited mountain gardens on vacations. She continued to entertain, to build meals on vegetables, fruits, cheeses, fish, lamb, chicken —homegrown, fresh, organic, natural. Preservatives, beyond salt, and chemicals as coloring or additives were unknown to her.

Like most tourists with a bit of pull with officials, Kegan and I, and the Apissons on several of their many trips, tried to arrange to meet Shirali Mislimov. Living in the Republic of Azerbaijan near the Iranian border, Mislimov was reputed to be the oldest man in the world. He was 178 years old when he died quietly in September 1973. For some time, due to his frail condition, only blood relatives were permitted to visit him. We were unsuccessful in our efforts, but I have many notes on the man who was so unique that, at 168, a postage stamp was issued in his honor.

From my notes on Mislimov, I can report that his diet was basically the Caucasus diet we want you to adopt or adapt for your health and your family's.

A 157-year-old great-great-grandmother was the oldest "find" of our trip. She was very feminine, neatly groomed, another excellent culinary artist and very capable at helping the children with their schoolwork. Impatient when our questioning began to tax her by its length, she cut it short by exclaiming to her daughter, "They're starting to make me old. I see my first gray hair."

Garabed, another lively gentleman, was 127 years old. He was pleased to meet a delegation from Ameri*cahhh* and was impatient for us to meet his children. While we waited for them, he told us the legend of *herissah,* the traditional chicken-wheat porridge.

Garabed said that a zealous monk, weary from his day's labors, dozed off, forgetting to remove from the lowering fire his already much-stirred food for the next day. It cooked all night long, reaching the heavenly smoothness and thickness that characterizes this dish. When he awoke and tasted his accidental creation, he shouted in pleasure, "*Herissah,*" the local version of Hallelujah, by which name the concoction has been known ever since.

Garabed's children were soon present and properly admired. A ninety-year-old guest arrived and joined the conversation. He was duly toasted and, in his turn, toasted the "youngsters." He said, "Not since Dumas *père et fils* have we met such a succession of masters in the storytelling art."

Our 127-year-old host, Garabed, applauded with a dig. "I see you're a man of high literary acumen," he acknowledged. "But your mathematics is off. This boy of ninety summers, married a year ago and a new father, is not my son, but my grandson."

One day when Kegan was to meet a distinguished agricultural botanist, a centenarian near the botanist's home offered a repast for the American visitors. We sped into the highlands with our Russian entourage for the day's activities.

Our route took us past uranium deposits, we were told, and fields of grass-tuft and green herbs where the grazing sheep had glistening gold-plated teeth. If they ever unlock that secret of nature, dentistry could disappear.

We counted twenty-nine hairpin curves—navigated much faster than I enjoyed—from Lake Sevan, the top of the local world, near the mountains that have my husband's name, Kegan (Kerama Lehr), on a road that went hurtling down into a hidden valley. Leaving the road at a woolens plant where a secret process, they said, produces men's suiting materials from waste rock, we took little byroads past lovely private gardens and finally, six hours into nowhere, reached the enchanted cottage.

A ceremonial table awaited us. Our centenarian hostess did us proud with sheep (*karnoug*) kabob. Some items we ate that day bear description. One was *madzoon,* concentrated yogurt from sheep's milk, cut with a knife and eaten with a fork. Delicious. And we had a great variety of vegetables, cooked fresh as we shall tell you how to cook them, green salads, *bulgur* wheat to accompany the kabob, and for dessert, plates of breadstuffs. The breadstuffs were served with two kinds of honey, one whipped white, the other so thick that it was also cut with a knife and eaten with a fork.

Toasts by and for everyone present, as well as for many not present, were frequent and a challenge to our endurance. An enormous assemblage crowded into the cottage. Somehow there was food and drink for all. When I began taking pictures, our 100-plus hostess ran to fetch her husband to pose with her, snuggling up close to him on their porch.

An amazing woman, she produced that prodigy of food in a tiny kitchen, organized to the standards of a gourmet restaurateur. She brought her water in from an outdoor well. When I grew curious as to the whereabouts of the toilet, she ran me to the outhouse, where the floor was neatly sawed and one squatted.

When Kegan's botany business ended, our party raced back past a wild silver-black fox farm, a rarity in the world of fancy furs.

I have spared you most of the details of our travelogue because, though fascinating to us, they are not the purpose of this book. Now let me summarize as briefly as I can what we observed that *is* important to you concerning the healthy spirits and bodies of Caucasus elders we met, examined and interviewed.

Three months is not a lifetime. But I have added my own observations to those of the Apissons on their seven visits, and to twenty-five years of private practice, earlier nutritional work and an active role in our laboratory research. I offer my findings as food for thought and thought for food.

The reports on the habits and life spans of centenarians in other parts of the world have been subjected to severe questioning. But enough documentation exists in the Caucasus by way of living centenarians-plus to suggest that there, at least, something is taking place which Americans should know about and, as far as possible, imitate.

You see, the Caucasus diet works. Those hardy, vital people, one fourth of whole villages as we have said, are not merely centenarians because of the way they nourish themselves and exercise their bodies—they are productive centenarians, useful centenarians, glad they are alive because age has not proved an impediment to purpose and fulfillment. That is remarkable and that is what we hope to reveal to you as this book unfolds.

Yes, the ages of long-lived people in places like Hunza or Vilcabamba, Ecuador, have been attacked. Contrary to human nature elsewhere, these people are accused of *exaggerating* their ages or, at best, being mixed up about them, since official birth records are questionable or nonexistent.

I'm unconcerned over whether a man who says he's 127 has added a few years or if a woman of 105 says she's only 99 out of vanity. In the Caucasus, the government pensions off its elders on retirement. Governmental and church records are exact and clear. Not only do these people not exaggerate their ages, since the record would expose them, but they are too easily embarrassed by the available truth when they try to make themselves out younger than they are.

Even so, I have to tell you about one notorious practice among elderly Caucasus widowers. When wife hunting in the region, men in their high nineties, and especially those over a hundred, lie brazenly to the women they court. Even at those ages, women want *men* and are suspicious that one might be becoming deficient in sexual performance by the age of 100 or thereabouts.

Many of these late Caucasus marriages and remarriages quickly produce offspring, for a real incentive exists to prove manhood in advanced years and even a Caucasus centenarian knows he may not have much more time to prove the point.

No, I do not worry about those who might doubt ages which are confirmed by reliable records. To an American visitor, the evidence of the eyes is all-persuasive. Everywhere you look in that part of the world, you see people of well-advanced years with their large families, three and four generations, even the eldest full of vigor, full of humor, full of joy. Their numbers and vitality are living proof that the Caucasus diet works better for them than anything else on earth is working for us.

It's hardly farfetched for gerontologists in the U.S.S.R. to speculate on the human ability to reach 200 years when their Mislimov reached 178. On the whole, our medicine, plumbing and creature comforts of every kind are superior to theirs. Even so, I am obliged to offer you a regimen like theirs as the only way I know on earth to give you hope of 100 healthy, happy years.

Survival, these people have taught us, is a lifelong obligation and art form based on nutrition without chemistry. In our country today, against a mean array of induced dangers to health, survival demands a return to the natural way of our ancestors, the way by which they brought mankind into this century. I invite you to learn how to have your own Caucasus diet without moving there. It's in the chapters ahead.

3.

Fad Diets: Why You Should Avoid Them

Our American marketplace is saturated with diet books. They promise quick results and even deliver them for a while, but at what are increasingly recognized as high medical risks. I do not want to condemn them with one broad brush. However, I'd like to offer a few reasoned comments on popular fad diets in this chapter. At the same time, I am very anxious for you to understand that our Caucasus diet is not one of them.

The Caucasus diet, even our weight-off version which appears in Chapter 10, is not a starvation diet. I have never been able to understand why anyone should be persuaded to go on a starvation diet. Half the world starves, but not because it wants to diet. When medical teams examine the emaciated bodies of victims of starvation, they find anemia, bone-marrow disorders, serious infections, disease after disease. Does that picture suggest that *voluntary* starvation is a safe way to relieve obesity? Obviously not.

The Caucasus diet is also not an eat-what-you-please diet. How can that possibly solve a fat person's difficulties? Eat-what-you-please binges are what make most fat people obese in the first place.

Something else you don't see much of in the Caucasus is the philosophy of eat-what-you-please, you'll exercise it off. Plenty of exercise is available there, but most people just naturally limit themselves scrupulously on food.

Consider our government's findings on Korean and Vietnam GI's. These soldiers exercised as we at home never do, slogged in mud, taxed their bodies severely in swamp and jungle. Post-mortems on many of these young men revealed cardiovascular diseases, with evidence of fatty and hardened arteries. Evidently, no amount of exercise was capable of retarding the deterioration. I believe these youths needed far more attention to their diets than those in less physically taxing warfare.

My husband and I did not see all-protein and water diets in the Caucasus. With or without excess water flooding and flushing the system, evidence shows all-protein diets can be dangerous to the kidneys. People with weak kidneys, and even many who start with healthy kidneys, can develop gout, arthritis, diabetes and organ damage from heavy protein and water assaults on their systems.

Caucasus people avoid both excessive protein and too little. Some instinct has taught them that enough protein, but not too much, is necessary for healthy minds, muscles, bones, hearts and years. There is ample evidence that prolonged periods of low-protein dieting cause the body to recycle whatever protein it finds within itself. Carried on long enough, that process can be fatal.

Pot-bellied victims of kwashiorkor, a vitamin-deficiency disease found in children and infants that is common in underdeveloped countries but not unknown here, are found to lack vital amino acids. The disease brings on diarrhea, fatty infiltration of the liver, apathy, atrophy of muscles and other symptoms. Unrelieved, it is fatal. No, don't starve yourself of proteins to lose weight. There's a safer way.

The Caucasus diet is not Zen-like or macrobiotic. I don't attack vegetarian diets as such, but macrobiotic diets in this country have caused fatalities.

That brings us to fatty diets. Caucasus plateau and highland folk raise animals as they raise themselves—lean. They do not fatten animals for marketing purposes, so their meats are less fatty. Whatever fat does appear in food preparation is painstakingly trimmed away.

We should do the same. Since we are bombarded with cuts of deliberately market-fattened meat, we should just as deliberately seek out the leaner cuts and refuse to buy the product untrimmed. That might discourage the sweet souls whose jobs consist of figuring out new ways to add more lard to the content of our cuts.

A side benefit of eliminating meat fats would be a drop in our national tendency toward heart disease, hardening of the arteries, high blood pressure, strokes and diabetes, occurring even in our children. All these are increasingly being linked to high ingestion of animal fats, with excessive cholesterol suspected of a prime role in our susceptibility.

I do not want to give the impression that *selected* fats in our everyday diet are unimportant. Our Caucasus diet is not deficient or skimpy in the *right* fat values. Vitamins A, D and E and other nutrients come from vegetable fats. Diets omitting or cutting too far back on proper (heavily but not entirely vegetarian) fats have produced skin abnormalities, infections, poor hair conditions, poor physiques and shortened lives in test animals and people. Among these studies are my own, convincing me that a nonfat diet is another road to suicide if carried on long enough.

The Caucasus diet is also not too low in carbohydrates. Contrary to some currently popular fad diets, the health-survival regimen of Caucasus centenarians includes carbohydrates (and a subdivision called fiber that we'll talk about later) from unrefined whole-grain cereals, grasses, sprouts, vegetables and fruit.

Now let's run down the don't diets again by some of their names, bad diets all. You probably have some on your bookshelves: the meat and water diet, bananas and milk diet, milk diet, half-grapefruit diet, water diet, juice diet, sixty-gram carbohydrate diet, zero-gram carbohydrate diet. I hate them all. I see them demineralizing you, creating deficiencies, being destructive to your sex organs and capability, harmful to body, soul, mind and spirit. Especially if prolonged, they are frontal attacks on normal youth, body chemistry, creativity, color, faculties, tissue resilience, organs.

Meat and Water Diet

Weight comes off, but at what expense and for how long? Wolfing down big fat-marbled steaks, you consume injurious quantities of animal fat. The chicken and mayonnaise diet is an equal offender. I see bodies dangerously overloaded with cholesterol, which can clog arteries with hormones harmful in steady large increments and with dangerous amounts of saturated fat.

And what's *not* in the meat and water diet is just as dangerous as what is in it. Where is your vitamin B_6 supply? Any that is found in the meat is destroyed by braising. Where are the minerals you require? Not in braised meat. Where is the natural fiber count? None. Suppose you take vitamin supplements. All that water in a meat and water diet, without balancing nutrients, just flushes the vitamins and minerals away. At the same time, you're overloading and threatening your kidneys.

If your kidneys weren't 100 percent healthy to start with, this is a dangerous flirtation. The absence of fruit, grains and vegetables doesn't let you get your quota of vitamins and minerals naturally, which might help you tolerate the diet to a better extent.

I believe the variations—chicken only, turkey only, fish only, shellfish only, the egg diet, *any* mono-diet—are dangerous. What saves most of us is that we get bored or discouraged before there's permanent damage.

Low- or Zero-Carbohydrate–High-Calorie Diet

As a physician and researcher, I find such an approach, not for a day or week but forever, unthinkable. For many who try it, forever may prove far shorter than anticipated. What's wrong with it? It's unnatural and deficient. You gobble heavy cream, butter, mayonnaise, cheeses, meats, fish and fowl, but no fruits, no grains, no vegetables, no cereals. The permitted half-cup of shredded lettuce is removed quickly if weight loss isn't forthcoming, whereupon you're advised to meet that unnatural condition with laxatives. Caucasians don't need laxatives even though—poor, healthy primitives—many still squat in outdoor facilities.

Honestly, how do you imagine that glut of meat, solid animal fat, butter-and-eggs routine for life will affect your intestines? Your once-in-a-lifetime heart? Your one and only body? Your God-given impulses and sexual performance? Can it give you an eye that twinkles and marvelous desire for another wife in your nineties? No, whatever time it gives you will not afford you or your wife much pleasure. Fortunately, you're likely to be bored to death before you're done to death. But why take the chance?

Why wait until you reach bloat plateau, where even the weight loss that temporarily made the diet look good stops? Why wait until your hands are puffy, your skin discolored, your eyes fishy and watery looking, your arteries a bit more hardened? How in heaven's name can deliberately induced deficiencies make people healthy, young and beautiful? And what becomes of your temper, your personality, your peace of mind?

Juice Diets

These diets, too, do not meet the total needs of your body. Where are your protein sources? The dangerous answer is, *you* become your protein source. As we have said, the body draws on itself for protein, soon depriving its bone and muscle tissue, making the body susceptible to disease. Another problem, of course, unless all juice is fresh and full of pulp, is that the diet supplies absolutely no fiber!

Bananas and Milk Diet

This is another defective diet, lopsided in a different way—far overweighted with carbohydrates. Where are the vital minerals, proteins, iron, vitamins? Not there. I've seen people brought in as emergency hospital patients from trying to limit their weight this way.

Sixty-Gram Carbohydrate Diet

The body needs carbohydrates, fewer than sixty grams as a rule, on a daily basis. Surrounding the right number should not be Hollandaise sauce, custards, whips and toppings, sugary starches and starchy sugars, empty puddings and pies, cream soups, wines and the like.

I hope you have gathered by now that *no* diet which fails to supply the body's continuous basic needs *from day to day* is anything to fool with. If your doctor recommends taking weight off, it should be accomplished without neglecting your bones as well as those fat deposits, your organs, tissues, veins and arteries—your total self. Fad diets fail you in this important way, but, as I have promised you, the Caucasus diet is not one of them.

Grapefruit Diet

By now you can recite its deficiencies. Where are the proteins? What happens to bones and muscles deprived of proteins? Remember, just getting thinner isn't enough. Everywhere in the world, people who have starved to death because they were unable to get food have proved that point often enough to spare you such a diet.

No Citrus Diet

This diet excludes them all—oranges, lemons, limes, grapefruit, citron, and so on. And no milk or bread, either. The dieter "compensates" with some eighty-seven pills a day. A fishbowl is filled with them and the dieter grabs a fistful whenever he thinks of it. The prime advocate of this diet is no longer among us. I hope not too many others have been taken away. This is a dangerous diet, deficient, defective. Don't.

Three-Day Prune Diet

This is similar to the no-prune diet; egg diet; raw vegetables and/or fruit and egg diets; four-eggs-a-week diet; no-eggs diet; meat and suet, all-meat, little-meat and no-meat diets. People self-prescribe such diets in endless variations. To sum them all up, there is no gain in trading existing poor food habits for a freaky new set.

Survival rule: Never let a diet tempt you because it sounds exotic. Like the alleged balm of Zen, when Americans try to imitate it, usually badly, it may be more deadly than beneficial.

Our Caucasus diet is not exotic. Some of the dishes, when we use their foreign names, may sound enticingly different. But you'll find that the basic foods are very familiar.

But don't let our *un*dramatic basics fool you. It's time you shed your susceptibility to every new fad coming down the road and got back to nature's ways. Our diet sustains and lengthens life. Our reducing diet, with its balanced limitations, will take weight off safely. It's all you need if you're not beyond nature's help.

Now I'm going to cite a case history. There will be others

later. This one is inserted not as a success story but to explain something you must know—that we are all physically and chemically individuals and that no one pat solution can possibly work equally for all. There must be variations, subtleties that we learn to apply to ourselves to make the broad principles work best.

The case history I want to tell you about is Morvyth McQueen-Williams, a medical doctor whose exposure to Herbert McLean Evans and Kegan Sarkisian awoke in her a great interest in Caucasus diet secrets.

As a result of this interest, am I a slip of a woman, at ideal body weight, the living example of what can be accomplished with a Caucasus diet? No, I am large-framed and not since my years at Johns Hopkins have I been at ideal body weight. During those years, this body I carry around with me was severely damaged by radiation pollution not yet sufficiently understood or feared by us in those years. I have needed and, with my husband's help, have had available to me much more than the diet I shall recommend to hold my own against periodic flareups of radiation sickness which will shorten my years.

Johns Hopkins was a great adventure for a young doctor. In June 1941, I was house officer at that great medical school hospital complex. For four fantastic years I was part of the tradition of Sir William Osler, Drs. Howard Atwood Kelly, William Stewart Halsted and William Henry "Popsy" Welch, the big four of Hopkins' golden era. Hopkins was the envy of the world, surpassing Europe's best clinics. Presidents and kings joined the impoverished as patients, the wealthy nearly paying for free services to the poor. All received the same thorough testing and services.

At Hopkins I saw realized the ideals of my two heroes, Dr. Herbert Evans and Dr. Harvey Cushing. The staff worked around the clock, sacrificing themselves, bleary-eyed from night emergencies after heavy day schedules. In four years I never heard a complaint as the staff dwindled under the demands of World War II.

Going-away parties were frequent as the able-bodied doctors squeezed themselves into the original, and then a second, "Hopkins Unit." Some we toasted and feted never returned. Demands on the remaining staff doubled and redoubled, taking tolls on those of us who stayed behind.

It was as exhausting as it was exciting. The famous and to-be famous of our era came and left in a never-ending parade. We met Dr. Perrin Long's pioneering research group, working twenty-four hours a day to produce penicillin on the premises. We consulted with Dr. Alfred Blalock, surgeon-in-chief, blue-baby pioneer with his great surgical team. Dr. Walter Dandy, head of two Hopkins neurosurgical teams, was in my consulting rooms daily. I worked with Dr. Edwards Park and L. Emmet Holt, two dear nutritionist colleagues published frequently in texts and articles on our favorite topics.

Hopkins' stream of medical greats included Chief Pathologist William G. MacCallum; Dr. Arnold B. Rich of tuberculosis fame; Drs. I. Ridgeway Trimble, George G. Finney, W. Halsey Barker; Merrill Sosman, who could easily have been our century's leading radiologist, a recent cancer victim; and many more I should mention, all treasured associations.

Radiation exposure in X-ray work was a bigger problem than we knew. The large rubber-lead protective aprons we wore were designed for males. My sagging apron left a contour along the nipple line exposed continually to radiation.

To my knowledge, only Dr. Sosman (cancer) and Dr. Manfred Guttmacher (leukemia) have succumbed. But numerous tumor growths, as well as local hair loss and skin manifestations, surfaced among other members of the Hopkins staff. We were exposed not only above our aprons, but also at thigh height, where the body manufactures its marrow. Unhappily, the book has not yet closed on damage and death to doctors in the Hopkins years. As I have told my collaborators of this book, I have had ample reason to include myself in the probable toll ultimately taken by those years.

I am not suggesting that our group at Hopkins was especially martyred. Radiation danger and damage turned up elsewhere, too, as galloping cancers, aplastic anemia and leukemia, to name the worst.

Orthopedic specialists set fractures and check bone alignment under radiation risk even to this day. Medical men in emergency rooms still run these risks, as do cardiologists and pediatric specialists using X-rays to check human hearts and doctors who remove foreign bodies. That's not all. Doctors who inject, as in pyelograms, angiography and dye placings, share these dangers.

Conditions have improved since the early forties. But there will always be times when, unable to flee behind a barrier, the doctor has to stand his ground and accept these radiation hazards as part of his work.

Dangerously as we lived, we were better off than those in the 1895–1930 era when the hands of personnel were severely burned. And such improvements as television screens for viewing amplified portions of the human body, replacing older, less safe equipment, were years away. I have to write that, in some places, the old, unsafe equipment is still in use today.

Monitoring for radiation levels is no complete answer. We

wore sensitivity badges by the end of the Hopkins period. Physicists occasionally dropped in for a look. But radiation pollution can act like much of the chemistry in the food we've been complaining about—the destruction can take years, even decades, to appear.

Kegan knew I was living on borrowed time. He turned his attention to developing mixtures of herbs and botanical derivatives for me that, we felt, would postpone as long as possible the effects of X-ray exposure. We have had more than a fair measure of success for a considerable number of patients as well as for myself, but I live with strong evidence that this frame around me is a frail vessel.

Recognizing that this subject is controversial, I maintain that Kegan's knowledge and devotion provided me with extra years to accomplish useful purposes with my training and that we have helped others similarly.

I have survived long enough to absorb and appreciate a natural approach to nutrition. I was fortunate enough to see acted out in the Caucasus the validity of organic diet and to develop a great sense of the urgency for people to turn back to living food while there is still time.

Keep this in mind as you apply our reasoning to yourself. Undamaged bodies have more resiliency than damaged ones. You have heard that people who stop smoking on time are capable of repairing discolored lung tissue from within. Likewise, those who turn to proper nutrition while still basically capable of repair—and that's most of you—can do as much for their entire bodies.

We're going to start you down the right road in the next chapter by getting you to know your needed nutrients, how much you need (when we know) and where the nutrients come from. I make you this promise: your careful and repeated reference to the next two chapters will, if you heed what you read, bring you longer, healthier years and more pleasure in everything you do to fill them.

4. Nutrients We Must Have: Vitamins

Please read this chapter and the next carefully—no skipping. Get to *know* your vitamins and minerals and the foods you find them in. Re-read and consult these two chapters as often as necessary until you have really mastered their basic nutritional information. Your thorough grasp of the nutrients we must have and their best food sources are your threshold to better, longer life.

Wherever I can, I indicate from the best available data and my own experience what quantities of vitamins and minerals I believe are useful in supplementation of the daily diet. I want to emphasize that my recommendations will be for the AVERAGE ADULT and that they cannot apply equally to all, ESPECIALLY CHILDREN. Vitamin and mineral supplementation for infants and children cannot safely be read in a book and *must* be at your physician's discretion based on his knowledge of the children. Take this very seriously. Unthinking vitamin overdosage of young children can be fatal.

You may have gathered by now that it's my professional opinion that prolonged nutritional deficiency is the reason for most poor health and shortened life. Weather changes, germ and bacillus attacks, polluted air, abnormal exertion and/or periods of emotional stress find millions of us without reserves, suffering repeated illnesses because of nutritional deficiency.

When we're sick, prescribed medication can cause temporary chemical changes in us. Because of these changes, just when our bodies are struggling to overcome illness we may find ourselves craving more food than we need, thereby overeating and stuffing our systems. Weight rises, body balance is out the window and we plunge right backwards with a relapse.

Or, just as bad, illness depresses the appetite. We pop pills, scuttle body balance by pouring in liquor and other stimulants, and sink back into prolonged sickness, deficiency, sexual inadequacy and shortened lives.

It's no new observation that poor eating habits cause us trouble. For centuries, sailors sickened and died during long sea voyages. Finally, we learned that death of scurvy (vitamin C bankruptcy) can come from prolonged absence of fresh fruits and vegetables from the diet.

In the Crimean War, 25,000 French soldiers died of malnutrition, not battle. Scurvy, not bullets, killed 15 percent of those who died in our Civil War.

My own cases and others I have read of show that recovery from illness is often aided by prodigious quantities of vitamins and minerals. More and more today we hear about megavitamins, doctor-supervised massive vitamin dosing. In my experience, once full health is restored, massive dosing is best stopped in most cases. This is certainly true for my patients who have come to understand and live by better nutrition.

Freshness of food is vital to how nutritious it really is. How you cook it also decides how nutritious it is when it reaches your mouth. Pouring cooking water down the drain probably deprives you of most of your water-soluble vitamins.

Stale food may be worthless and dangerous to health. Heavy toasting robs bread of food values, assuming they are there in the first place. The truth is, you may be roasting, steaming, toasting or pouring away nutrients you think you're getting. If you have never thought about that, chances are you're a victim of the habit. The only consolation I can offer is that this is probably happening in the best of households.

Since few urbanites can buy enough fresh food, and because personal preparation methods further shortchange many of us, I recommend to my patients *moderate* vitamin/mineral supplementation. I will go into that as we move along. And I have charted average adult recommendations at the end of Chapter 5, which is on minerals.

It's often claimed that synthetic supplements are as good as those from natural sources. I doubt it. There can be differences, for instance, between liquid concentrates of soy, liver, natural whole fruit or vegetable preparations and pills available to supply the same ingredients synthetically. As a rule, liquids are better absorbed, and they excel especially when prepared as vitamin and mineral combinations.

Through necessity, there are exceptions. In pantothenate,

it's hard if not impossible to get all you need every day in natural food or form. A pantothenate pill can be a vital necessity. Also, people allergic to citrus, tomatoes, strawberries, wheat, eggs and the like go to synthetic supplementation with complete justification.

Now, the basics I want you to learn:

VITAMIN A

The average adult needs 7,000–10,000 International Units a day. Many of us cannot absorb that much; we vary greatly. As much as 10,000 units is five times the Recommended Dietary Allowance (RDA). You should get most of your vitamin A through careful attention to diet. But even when your diet contains the foods supposedly supplying enough vitamin A, to insure against this vitamin's depletion through staleness, cooking errors or whatever else may befall your purchases, supplement modestly with 4,000 units a day (for adults), no more.

Vitamin A is abundant in nature. It's in our green and yellow vegetables—most when freshest. It's in yellow-colored fruits—the richer the color the more A. It's in cantaloupe, honeydew, yogurt, liver, cultured milk, cream (use sparingly, for other reasons), butterfat (use sparingly); apricots, carrots, broccoli, romaine, chard, beet greens, spinach, collards, celery, squash; fish roe, fish liver, swordfish, smelts, salmon and many other fish. Botanicals rich in vitamin A are mint, parsley, green nuts, alfalfa, watercress, seaweed, green herbs, chicory, endive and dandelion. Other good sources are okra, unpared cucumbers, green asparagus, green peppers, chick-peas, deep-colored yams, sweet potatoes, beans, sprouts; chicken livers, kidneys, eggs, wheat germ and cheeses.

With so many sources, you can avoid any that disagree with you and still meet your daily needs with the supplementation I have suggested. The list of vitamin-A sources shows that, to take advantage of nature's bounty, it's smart to get over childhood hatreds of liver, cod-liver oil and fresh vegetables.

How badly do we need vitamin A? My work with rats proved that without it, males can't sire offspring and females become sterile. Vitamin A promotes sound teeth, bones, skin, eyes and hair; and it helps combat infection, especially of the epithelial tissue, as in the mouth. Vitamin A assists growth and strengthens our immunity systems.

The Caucasus diet is very high in vitamin A. And we found there fertility to advanced ages, normal livers and very little cancer. Is there a connection between healthy livers and freedom from cancer? I have seen evidence of that. Prolonged vitamin-A deficiency may play a role in cancer susceptibility. Lack of vitamin A can damage the liver, decreasing the organ's ability to form vital enzymes. Without enzymes, the body can't rid itself of estrogens and has difficulty detoxifying chemicals and throwing off poisons, as is the case in normal metabolic breakdown. The French forever concern themselves with their livers, and we should, too.

On this same point I've seen vitamin A applied, medically supervised, to skin cancers with beneficial results.

Vitamin A isn't the only liver-protecting vitamin. The B vitamins in very large doses sometimes correct pronounced liver damage. Research has shown, too, that vitamin B_6 plays a role in prevention of bladder cancer.

Vitamin A is oxidized—destroyed—by overcooking. Use pots that can be covered tightly with lids. Use *little* water. Cook as lightly as possible and just before serving. Learn to eat more raw fruits and vegetables (see Chapter 9 on fiber!). Don't braise liver to leathery worthlessness or the A will be wasted. Don't leave milk products on your doorstep too long—light destroys vitamin A. For the same reason, keep your vitamin-A tablets and capsules away from light. Buy perishables *fresh* (if they're wilted, they're stale) in small quantities for quick use, and then buy again. Storage, even frozen, wastes vitamin A along with other vitamins and minerals.

We benefit more from vitamins and minerals taken in combinations. For example, taken together, vitamins A and E strengthen one another's benefits. Barbara Apisson reminds us that food habits of the Caucasus show an instinctive rudimentary knowledge of this fact. Bulgur, Barbara points out, is habitually taken with a few teaspoonfuls of yogurt. Thus, amino acid and vitamin values combine and reinforce one another when single Caucasus meals combine grains, seeds and grain oils with vegetables, yogurt and animal proteins—a natural way of combining vitamins for extra yield.

Peoples in the Caucasus have been eating that way for centuries. Try it. In planning meals, mix. In regular diets, a few teaspoonfuls of yogurt or the same amount of any animal protein balances out lacks in grains, peas, lentils, chick-peas, bread, corn or potatoes. Don't overeat through combinations, but increase your food values by combining small quantities of more foods.

VITAMIN B_1

This vitamin is also called *thiamine*. It's best to get as much vitamin B_1 as possible directly from nature. But be warned—with vitamin-B deficiency affecting one out of every five people in the United

States, and with the cost of getting it from animal sources straining our budgets, we plainly must look past our supermarkets for its supply. Try to keep that in mind when we discuss the physical and practical benefits you can get from gardening in Chapter 8.

Vitamin B_1, the pep vitamin, is available in yogurt, yeast, wheat germ, whole wheat, barley, whole grains, sprouts, seeds, wild rice and potatoes; lean meat, liver, heart, brain and organ meats, in general; mussels, oysters and fish roe; and peas, beans and almonds.

Do not oversoak or overcook vitamin-B_1 foods. Again, use little water in cooking, cook lightly and don't throw the water away. Consume your cooking water—most likely your B_1 is in it, too. Use it in cooking or chill and drink.

Many herbs and botanicals are additional B_1 sources. That includes most herbal greens, such as parsley, mint, dandelion greens, watercress and mustard greens particularly. To learn more, get books on wild foods and edible weeds. Use them to learn to recognize the edibles and pick them where and when you can. Join garden clubs. They'll teach you to recognize such nutrients as the wild-growing but very common lamb's-quarters, rich in both vitamin B_1 and carotene. Carotene is provitamin A, which simply means it's a substance your body chemistry turns into vitamin A.

Most fruits, except for wild berries, have little vitamin B_1. Another B_1 food is dulse, coarse reddish seaweeds that also contain calcium and iodine, important minerals. For more natural B_1, meet bladderwick, kelp and fenugreek, as well as romaine and other edible lettuces and, certainly, nutritional yeasts described below (not baking yeast which, eaten uncooked as food, makes people gassy).

Brewer's yeast can vary in vitamin-B_1 content from 1 milligram (mg.) + per tablespoon to much more. Read the labels. Yeast flakes furnish up to 2.4 mg. of vitamin B_1 per tablespoon. Torola yeast can provide as much as 3.5 mg. of B_1. Nutritional yeasts also provide good amounts of niacin, pantothenic acid and vitamin B_6—in all, some dozen members of the B complex. If you can't stand the taste of B-rich nutritional yeasts or drown them in other foods, supplementation may have to be the way to get enough B_1.

Here's a suggestion: In the Caucasus, Barbara Apisson recalls for us, local malts, germinated from barley grains, are a good source of vitamin B_1. Caucasus beers, like most European beers, ferment slowly without sugar and are less bloating than U.S. beers, which are quick-fermented with as much as 10 percent sugar added. For those not concerned about weight, imported beer may provide another option.

Getting back to ordinary baking yeast, there are reports that it sets up an action in the intestines that can *deprive* users of vitamin B_1. Again, don't confuse it with nutritional yeasts.

I recommend 2 mg. of thiamine (B_1) a day as a supplement, which is twice the Minimum Daily Requirement (MDR).

Prolonged use of purgatives, antibiotics and other drugs can interfere with B-complex flora. Minimize this danger with yogurt between doses. And try to avoid prolonged dosing of any medicines. If you have been on anything for a while, check with your doctor about when to stop. You may find that he intended you to taper off or quit much sooner. Worse mischief than vitamin-B_1 imbalance can result from unnecessary and unintended prolonged (or combined) drug dosing.

VITAMIN B_2

This vitamin is also called *riboflavin*. I usually suggest 2.5 mg. a day as supplementation for my patients. To repeat an important warning, all doses I'm suggesting are AVERAGE ADULT. For children and infants, *vitamin supplements should be administered strictly under doctor's orders*. As I have said, overdoses can harm or kill infants. Please never forget that fact.

Again, get all the vitamin B_2 you can from nature. You are if you are eating most of the foods mentioned for vitamins A and B_1: yogurt, liver, kidney, heart, mustard greens and wild greens, wheat germ, yeast, soybeans. You also get vitamin B_2 in broccoli, mushrooms, almonds and other nuts, seeds, fruits and botanicals like mustard greens, hickory nuts, parsley and lettuce.

Caution: Light destroys riboflavin, too. Protect foods and supplements from light. If your fresh food has been exposed, supplementation makes even more sense.

All the sources I quoted for thiamine also provide riboflavin. There is vitamin B_2 in yeast flakes or powder, wild rice, rice polishings, organ meats and dairy products. Vegetarians tend to have too little vitamin B_2. Unless they are particularly knowledgeable about vegetarian foods, they need B_2 supplements more than the rest of us.

VITAMIN B_3

This vitamin is also called *niacin*. I recommend adding 15 mg. a day to your diet. That's 1½ times the MDR. Vitamin B_3 is called the memory vitamin, B_2 the longevity vitamin and, as I said, B_1 the pep vitamin. Vitamin B_3 does seem to jog the memory in cases of mental illness and senility. Normal memories work better on it, too.

Vitamin B_3 occurs in bran, bran coverings of nuts, yeast, wheat germ, whole-grains, squash, barley, rice polishings, liver, chicken, brains, lamb, pork, tongue, sweetbreads, heart, kidneys, lean meat, nut butter, almonds, buckwheat, mushrooms, apricots, soy, broccoli, yogurt, melon, fish roe, and seafood, especially mussels, also haddock, herring and salmon. Like vitamins B_1 and B_2, B_3 is found in plant and animal tissues.

When niacin comes from plant foods, the body must change it to use it. When the pantothenic-acid level is deficient, niacin deficiency and a condition resembling pellagra can result. Niacin has emerged in orthomolecular medicine as a keystone in megavitamin therapy.

Niacin is important in combination with other B vitamins for brain performance, sugar-starch metabolism, tissue respiration and other body functions. It is sometimes prescribed in massive doses for heart conditions. I prescribe time-release niacin capsules (prescription dose: 400 mg. per capsule) for elderly mental and memory-loss cases. On two or three a day, patients have "good days." But there seems little or no carry-over. If dosing stops, patients tend to backslide immediately.

More niacin sources are mushrooms, fresh sunflower and sesame seeds, dried nuts or fruits, brown and wild rice, alfalfa, parsley, peas, beans, chard, herb seeds like burdock, fenugreek, garden greens, dandelions, lamb's-quarters, artichoke, asparagus, okra, rutabaga, watercress, sage and turnip greens.

VITAMIN B_6

This vitamin, also called *pyridoxine,* is known as the nerve vitamin. It seems to work best in combination with magnesium (see Chapter 5). Vitamin B_6 is involved with brain and protein metabolism. Without it, babies can have convulsions and die or be anemic. Its lack is also seen in heart cases, insomnia, tremors, and in toxemia of pregnancy. We mentioned that patients on antibiotics sometimes develop deficiencies. Once vitamin-B_6 deficient, they require large doses until balance is restored. Elderly alcoholics have been shown deficient in B_6, magnesium and potassium. And there are reports of severe vitamin-B_6 deficiency leading to symptoms of epilepsy and schizophrenia.

Dieters changing from low-protein to high-protein regimens need extra vitamin B_6 and magnesium to metabolize the extra protein. In sex-power loss, sometimes the problem is traced to a lack of B_6 in the pituitary gland.

Vitamin B_6 is found in wheat germ, wheat and other bran, rice polishings, whole grains, liver, kidney, heart, spleen, sweetbreads, oil of nuts or grains, molasses, honey and egg yolk.

I usually advise 3 mg. daily of vitamin B_6 for supplementation. It takes real know-how to get as much as 2 to 3 mg. in your food. Even then, up to 50 percent loss can come from overcooking, heat-charring (as with meats), or through overwashing or oversoaking. Vitamin B_6 is another water-soluble vitamin often poured off in the cooking water. In special cases, I prescribe up to 100 mg. a day as a supplement.

Pantothenate

This is another member of the B family. I put average daily need at the odd total of 36 mg., though researchers have not agreed on a formula. I'll explain my views on how much we need a day. Pantothenate is attached to and apparently a vital part of coenzyme A. The latter is an indispensable link in the remarkable chemistry that converts food into energy. One of the coenzyme's important jobs is tearing down consumed fat. And without pantothenate, adrenocortical hormones cannot be manufactured in the body.

Pantothenate foods are liver, kidney, heart, brain, yeast, wheat germ, sesame seeds, sunflower and other seeds, the non-oil fraction of most nuts and peanuts, yogurt, wheat bran, bulgur, whole-grain wheat, brown rice, rice polishings, lentils, peas, beans, soy, chick-peas, oats, mushrooms, egg yolks, salmon, flounder, sole, kale, cauliflower, broccoli, cabbage, turkey, chicken, chopped liver, queen bee jelly and molasses. Milk and eggs provide a good ratio, ten times as much pantothenate as vitamin B_1.

Dry heat destroys pantothenate. Toast breads minimally. I advise patients to throw away their toasters. Sorry G.E. and Westinghouse, but that's the way the pantothenate crumbles.

While we're offending, I'll add that refining flour and grain destroys pantothenate, too. Lack of pantothenate in the diet may lead to skin ulcers, loss of hair, premature graying and other deficiency evidences. (Shortages of copper, low-protein diets, PABA* deficiency, B-complex shortage and folic acid, riboflavin, biotin and carotene lacks all can contribute to raking hair from your scalp.)

Doctors prescribe large doses of pantothenate and vitamin B_1, in combination, for decline after the age of thirty, and in cases of

**See next vitamin in the B family.*

hypertension and arthritis. Large doses are also worth a try for improving sexual performance and to fight depression found in dietary deficiency. Extra pantothenate may be needed by patients on antibiotics as well as those under high stress and by athletes (for their muscles).

In human milk, the ratio of pantothenate to vitamin B_1 is about 18 to 1. I have a strong feeling that that ratio may well be an ideal one for people of all ages, young and old. However, for those under high stress, as for example athletes, I do not hesitate to recommend 100 mg. a day with a corresponding increase in vitamin B_1. Taking 36 mg. a day as I have recommended ought to work pretty well for most people who, like you and me, can never be sure how much pantothenate, vitamin B_1, or anything else effectively reaches us from day to day in our diets.

PABA

Also in the B family, PABA is short for para-aminobenzoic acid. No MDR or RDA exists for it. In fact, some authorities doubt that PABA is a vitamin, while others call it a vitamin within a vitamin because of its close kinship with folic acid, a B vitamin we'll come to a bit later. PABA is more plentiful than folic acid, which is needed to prevent anemia. In a pinch, our systems can convert the more plentiful PABA to folic acid, sometimes draining our hair of color to save our blood from becoming anemic.

Few commercial supplements include PABA and folic acid. If using one, take the trouble to look for both. Paba foods are liver, most organ meats and, in fact, most lean meats; yeast, bran including rice polishings, all nuts and seeds, whole-grain breads and cereals, wheat germ; and leafy green vegetables. Because of PABA's role as a folic-acid surrogate, and because of how hard folic acid is to get in nature, I have decided that 100 mg. of PABA is a sensible supplement for protective purposes.

Inositol

Inositol is also in the B family. The estimated daily need is 1,500-3,000 mg. As with PABA and pantothenate, inositol is considered a youth vitamin. The three together are sometimes effective in reversing gray hair. Test doses on balding mice grew complete hair coverings in three weeks.

Inositol appears important to healthy intestines. As is the case with choline, coming up next, inositol is a factor in reducing cholesterol and in slowing hardening of the arteries. The combination of inositol and choline is also beneficial to liver maintenance.

We find inositol and choline in lecithin and soy products. Your best food source for lecithin is sesame seed (*tahini*, a Caucasus staple). Brewer's yeast is the most common U.S. source of lecithin. Lecithin works best when taken at the same time as an unsaturated oil such as oil of nuts, seeds, fish or flaxseed, for emulsification. Take lecithin with breakfast, adding a teaspoon of unsaturated oil to your orange juice.

Those who scoff at lecithin as something faddists dreamed up should know about recent studies at the Simon Stevin Research Institute, Belgium, reporting marked lowering of lipids in the blood after two weeks of injection of soybean lecithin into 100 patients. Plasma cholesterol was lowered by 40 percent. There were other improvements in concentrations of low-density lipoproteins, which are known to play a role in a type of arteriosclerosis.

Other inositol sources are grapefruit, beef heart, brain, wheat germ, oranges, melon, blackstrap molasses and such legumes as chick-peas, peas, beans and lentils. Soybean lecithin contains about 5 percent inositol. Three tablespoons of brewer's yeast can provide 1,000 mg. of inositol, half a grapefruit as much as 500 mg.

For my patients with heart conditions, I usually prescribe three 19-grain (1,200-mg.) capsules a day of natural soybean lecithin, one taken with each meal. I often add large quantities of vitamin C-rich botanicals.

Hint: Heavy coffee drinkers are well-advised to take note of their need for extra inositol. Caffeine destroys it. People should get all the inositol they can. Coffee and cola addicts most likely need even more than the 3,000 mg. mentioned earlier.

Choline

Yet another member of the B family. I described choline as a youth vitamin. On the average, I suggest 1,500–2,000 mg. a day for supplementation. Some of us can absorb and benefit from as much as 3,000 mg. daily.

Choline, in conjunction with vitamin C, inositol and vitamin E, benefits the liver. High-fat and/or high-protein dieters—steak-, chop- and roast-lovers—should fortify themselves with this supplement group. In such diets, choline shortage can lead to elevated cholesterol levels. Alcoholics who skimp on solid foods and therefore nutrients chronically show up deficient in these life-support vitamins. Choline lack can also cause obesity, high blood pressure, heart disease, hardening of the arteries, weak kidneys and susceptibility to diabetes.

Choline food sources are yeast (three tablespoons of

brewer's yeast may provide as much as 1,050 mg. choline), liver, liver extract, heart, brain, kidney, sweetbreads—in fact, all the endocrines; egg yolks, fish roe, fish and poultry; soy, chick-peas, beans, peas, wheat germ, beet greens, mustard greens, turnip greens, spinach and whole grains.

To get choline in a supplement, I tell patients, take lecithin, especially if you're on a reducing diet trying to burn fat. You can sprinkle lecithin granules on foods, use them in cooking, sprinkle them on snacks and take one 4-grain tablet after breakfast and one 19-grain capsule after dinner. Never worry about lecithin. I've never heard of anybody getting too much.

Adequate daily choline helps prevent gallstones, sand or gravel. It is available in oil or granular form, in the B-complex group in liquid form, or as tablets or capsules. Lecithin is particularly important to older people whose hardened arteries can shorten their lives. When you realize that lecithin and the B complex also aid their memories, older persons plainly need and deserve such supplements.

Biotin

Another B vitamin, biotin is sometimes called the cheerful vitamin. Why cheerful? Because severe lack of biotin causes severe depression. The average adult need is 1 mg. a day.

Here's an oddity: People on otherwise fine diets can become deficient in biotin by eating many raw eggs. People on hurry-up pep meals of raw eggs, eggnogs and other freakish diets may become victims. Anyone with a strong raw-egg habit can stop losing biotin immediately by cooking the eggs. Or, you can cook the whites and eat the yolks raw if you want.

If you've been on a raw-egg kick, biotin supplementation is probably needed. But many vitamin formulas omit biotin. You need that 1 mg. a day. Make sure you get it. Always read your label.

The best food sources of biotin are liver, yeast, *cooked* eggs, cauliflower and most nuts and seeds. Others are fish roe, oysters, salmon; pork, beef, lean meats generally; corn, wheat germ and yogurt. Mushrooms contain some biotin, too. A three-ounce serving of beef liver is good for 1 mg. of biotin if cooked lightly.

Liquid dieters can avoid losing biotin by stirring eggs into hot soup. Eggs beaten slightly with lemon juice thicken soup without destroying biotin. Homemade mayonnaise, Hollandaise and other fancy sauces, should have only egg yolks in them. Get all the white out. Scrambled eggs should be thoroughly cooked, not loose and runny.

Folic Acid

Our next B vitamin, folic acid, helps build healthy red blood cells and bone marrow. The average daily adult need is 1 mg. Folic acid is not easily found and is rare in supplements. It is seldom found in nonprescription amounts higher than 100 micrograms (mcg.) or .1 mg.

This restriction was adopted to prevent pernicious anemia sufferers from masking their symptoms. Only doctors should manage pernicious anemia. To underscore, folic acid is the vitamin most lacking in American diets.

Folic acid deficiency can be dangerous. Human blood and bone marrow tests have shown damaged chromosomes resulting from folic acid and vitamin-B_{12} deficiency. Treating patients with folic acid, vitamin B_{12}, or both, corrected the problem.

Young pregnant women who are dieting to stay slim have sometimes been found lacking in folic acid. Figuring that anyone in such a state is probably shortchanging herself on other vitamins, too, doctors tend to treat these women with vitamin C and all the B vitamins, including folic acid.

Liver, which we've already seen is a nutrient storehouse, is our best source of folic acid. Folic acid also comes in asparagus, dark-green leafy vegetables, broccoli, Brussels sprouts, watercress, egg yolks, yogurt, cheese, almonds, peanuts, brown rice, wheat, oats, and, to a lesser degree, mushrooms. Small amounts of folic acid are also found in lettuce, romaine, endives, apricots, berries and tangerines. It's also present in coconuts, dates, avocados, sweet corn, cultured milk (buttermilk, kefir or tan made from yogurt) and sprouted seeds and beans. Add your sprouts to soup *after* cooking, eating them raw to avoid destroying folic acid. Eat them raw in salads, too.

As I said, folic acid, too seldom seen in vitamin-B formulas, comes in 100 mcg. or .1 mg. supplements. That small amount is usually enough to prevent dangers of folic acid deficiency.

Cobalamine (B_{12})

Cobalamine is the last presently identified vitamin in the B family.* One of the more recently studied, it has no MDR. Daily need has been estimated at .002 mg. or 2 mcg. I tell my patients to try to add 5 mcg. of B_{12} as a daily supplement, but the vitamin is not easy to find.

***At this writing, B_{15}, sodium pangamate, has appeared, is very new and is said to play a role in oxygen distribution in the blood. People report good results from its use, but not enough is known now for discussion.**

Vitamin B_{12}, like folic acid, is linked to healthy bone marrow, red blood cells and healthy minds. Stomach diseases, pernicious anemia and mental problems are sometimes traced to the body's inability to use vitamin B_{12} properly.

Vegetarians beware: Plants in this country have little vitamin B_{12}. Also, B_{12} is light-sensitive, water-soluble, and degenerates under acid or alkali excess. It not only helps maintain a healthy stomach, healthy nerves and bone, but helps metabolize fat. Those who need it most benefit more from injections than oral doses.

The richest sources of B_{12} are liver, kidney, cheese, yogurt, fish, fish roe, whole wheat, bulgur, whole-grain bread—and there's some in soy and eggs. Sea kelp is probably the best source of B_{12} for vegetarians.

VITAMIN C

This vitamin is an important antioxidant. Remember vitamin C, especially during our Chapter 9 discussion of antioxidants against diseases of the arteries. It is water-soluble and easily destroyed, and you need it daily because the body can't store it. During prolonged sweating, fever or stress, in any kind of illness, you most probably need extra amounts of vitamin C to normalize.

Because contact with copper destroys vitamin C, foods containing this vitamin should never be cooked in copper.

The MDR is 10 mg. for an infant, 20 mg. for one to twelve year olds and 30 mg. for an adult. I stand with the often-maligned forces who say this is simply not enough. Our bodies must have vitamin C for far too many important purposes to split hairs over it.

I have prescribed for myself and for adult patients as much as Linus Pauling suggests, for *short periods.* I *regularly* use and recommend no more than 500 mg. in time-release capsules for daily use of adults. It is clearer all the time that foods rich in vitamin C are vital to us, not only for the known reasons but to assist in many body functions whose daily needs we are still not clear about.

As the vitamin-C controversy continues, doctors continue to find C effective against exposure to pollutants such as DDT, cadmium and strychnine. They find it helps heal wounds and stomach ulcers. Recent work shows that a vitamin-C deprived liver cannot produce prothrombin, a substance which plays a role in coagulation of blood. Vitamin C's role in preventing scurvy with its often fatal damage to bones and joints is historical.

I'm also convinced that vitamin C promotes better body use of vitamins A, E, the B complex, iron, calcium and protein.

Many books have been written about vitamin C and health.

Vendettas have sprung up over it. There's far too much destructive vitamin-C politics in the health field. But I remember so unassailable a pillar of the establishment as Dr. Samuel C. Harvey, under whose guidance I did my Yale surgical thesis, writing on the wisdom of large doses of vitamin C plus protein in the preparation of patients for surgery. With existing research, both animal and human, down to the cellular and intracellular level, it is a jolt to see vitamin C's value still under attack.

I'm reminded of the work of Dr. Henricus J. Stander at Cornell. Women who miscarried frequently came to him from all over the world for treatment that included large doses of oranges and orange juice—with excellent results. In our own work with miscarriers, Kegan and I obtained similar results with extracts of vitamin-C rich herbs and botanicals.

The best sources of vitamin C are citrus fruits, tomatoes, green peppers, green vegetables, and most other fruits and vegetables. Always protect your purchases from light and heat. Vitamin-C rich foods should not be sliced until time of use. Alkalis as well as those copper utensils destroy vitamin C. Locally grown, fresh-picked produce is optimum for delivering C power to you before substantial loss.

Particularly for those who can't tolerate citrus, tomatoes or strawberries, and the rest of us, too, instead of wondering about how much vitamin C we're getting in our food—since C is so easily destroyed before we get it—add those 500 mgs. a day as a supplement and then eat only the C foods that agree with you.

In spite of those who say you get all you need in your diet and who can't know what they're talking about, the need for vitamin C is *constant*. We benefit most from low doses taken often or as available in time-release capsules.

Is the idea of often taking small amounts of vitamin C freakish? Not in this nation where we are popping candy, cookies, cigarettes and other useless-to-harmful things into our systems with fatalistic frequency during waking hours. Pop vitamin C instead of those empty foods—with breakfast, between meals, with lunch, dinner, at bedtime. Add it up to 500 mgs. when you're well, more when you're not.

VITAMIN D

This vitamin is *necessary*—for healthy teeth and bones, for childhood growth, for assimilation of calcium and other nutrients. Vitamin D works best when taken in combination with others. You get an efficient working mix in D plus vitamins A, E, K and F (in vegetable oils, for instance), and with vitamin C plus your minerals, especially calcium. The average adult diet requires 400 units a day. Like other fat-soluble vitamins, D is not sensitive to light but should be refrigerated to deter rancidity.

I'm impressed with the findings of Dr. Carl Reich and Dr. John Bennett of Canada that vitamin D in its natural state (not as a synthetic) has a role in the formation of hormonal substances and in the regulation of the blood calcium/phosphorus balance, thus extending D's influence beyond promoting healthy skeletal structure to the control of all muscle activity and functioning of all body cells.

The D vitamin formed beneath our skins when we expose our normally oily (unsoaped) surfaces to natural sunlight or ultraviolet from a lamp, the D in fish-liver oils and in such fish as smelts and sardines, eaten whole so that you get the liver, the D in fish roe and egg yolks—this natural vitamin D appears to be of benefit to a whole range of body functions only now beginning to be understood.

Information becoming available on how vitamin D synthesizes certain proteins and controls some hormone functions—giving D a part in cholesterol levels, among other vital functions—is persuading some authorities that D may really be a hormone, not a vitamin. And doubt is suddenly being cast on the effectiveness of fortifying foods by substances which can be irradiated for vitamin-D activity.

Synthetically irradiated vitamin D is known as D_2. The natural vitamin, found in the sources mentioned above, is classified as D_3. If you buy a supplement, caution suggests trying to get D_3 rather than D_2. Read your labels. Caution also dictates not overdosing children on vitamin D. At any age, too much D is a potential strain on the kidneys. But 400 units a day as a supplement is not excessive for adults, I am convinced.

We're learning much more about D. We'll all do well to keep D, vitamin or hormone, under scrutiny.

VITAMIN E

As health readers know, vitamin E remains controversial. In spite of being essential to daily life, sexual adequacy and longevity, nearly every claim about vitamin E will get you a strong argument. But on the basis of my work in E, I recommend 100 mg. a day as an average adult supplement.

It is no surprise to me that doctors are finally acknowledging that vitamin E somehow plays an important role in health. But people seeking improved sexual performance still hear their doctors call vitamin E controversial and prescribe instead psychiatric advice.

I know from my own experiments on animals that vitamin E is important to sexual performance.

The Evans research at Berkeley and work at many other laboratories has established that vitamin E exists in a great many unrefined and fresh foods. This has led some authorities to say that vitamin E supplements are a waste of money. It's not quite that simple. In daily life, the average U.S. diet is really very short on vitamin E in spite of the abundance of apparent sources. Let's examine why this is so.

Our animal sources provide us with a dribble of vitamin E. There is a little in fish roe, eggs, cream, fish, cheese, shark-liver oil, cod-liver oil, sardines, and the brains and livers of properly fed animals.

Except at health-food stores, plant sources like salad oils sell us short on vitamin E. The E that originally was in such sources is mostly removed and sold to fill the E-capsules people buy. And there is a ten-to-one likelihood that your lettuce has no vitamin E at all left in it by the time you buy it.

A little vitamin E is also contributed by beans. Soy is good if you have the time to soak and prepare the bean or eat the grits. There is vitamin E in green vegetables like leek; in the cabbage family, including Brussels sprouts; in herbs like dark-green fresh Italian parsley, dill, dandelion and cress. Having your own balcony box or home garden for growing these items fresh is a sane suggestion we'll make again in Chapter 8.

Fresh untoasted wheat germ may be available at local health-food stores. Some high-volume stores do get top quality, but it's scarce. If you do not live near such a store, you should buy supplements (capsules), store them in the refrigerator and take them with your multivitamins. And occasionally buy an eight-ounce bottle of unrefined, cold-processed raw wheat-germ oil, fresh from the Middle West, to store in the refrigerator and use up before too long. It comes sealed. It should not arrive rancid. One teaspoon of this oil provides about 10 international units (I.U.) of vitamin E. Taken with or between meals, that represents the oil value of five pounds of fresh whole wheat.

In animal or human adolescence, and especially with vigorous exercise, the need for vitamin E probably doubles. Sports teams that were experimentally put on vitamin E performed so much better that most athletes today take it. Team physicians recommend it even though doctors for nonathletes don't.

Foods rich in vitamin E abound in the Caucasus. It's in their walnuts, apples (extra vitamin E is extracted by chewing out the oils of apple peels and seeds), bulgur, whole grains, oils, greens, leeks and other fresh natural sources. We'll be smarter, too, to consume certain of our fresh fruits with their peels and seed pits.

Although our Berkeley experiments proved vitamin E's role in the sexual performance of animals, we are not concerned only with the lack of vitamin E in sexual performance. I learned from other experiments at Berkeley that vitamin-E deficiency can lead to an unhealthy nervous system, muscles, bone marrow, heart and truly a totally sick body.

At Berkeley we experimented in all the vitamins, but when it came to vitamin E, Dr. Evans led us in the classical workup of all time. We were guided step by step by this genius giant with his superabundant enthusiasm. Lights burned from dawn to 2:00 A.M. I know. Night after night I ran for the last train at that hour.

VITAMIN F

Though most charts omit it, you know vitamin F as *essential fatty acids,* important in sex-gland and prostate normality and needed for other glands, especially the adrenals. It is important in cardiovascular health, slowing cholesterol buildup; it promotes calcium availability to cells; it restores skin normalcy (preventing or helping correct eczema); and it fights asthma, sinus infections, common colds and allergies. Experiments show that vitamin F helps protect us from radiation, including X-ray damage.

Foods and botanicals containing essential fatty acids, the unsaturated-F values we need, are seeds, grains, nuts, green nuts and drupes (the walnut, almond and pine group especially provide vitamin F according to my own research). It also comes in vegetable and fish oils, if obtained by cold-pressing and eaten before they get rancid. Refining, improper exposure and storage all destroy vitamin F. So does hydrogenation, so common today in processed foods, as we've already griped.

Keep all F foods in dark containers in your refrigerator. Use minimum heating when cooking them. To get the vitamin F you need (there's no MDR or RDA for them), use vitamin-F foods generously, cook carefully and use plenty of F oils in your salads.

Mother's milk contains enough vitamin F within its linoleic, linolenic and arachidonic acids for baby's growth. Whole milk provides enough, too. Skim milk and skim-milk powders lack vitamin F but, unfortunately, they are used and even recommended. For vitamin-F safety, use whole milk, not skim or powdered! We know linoleic and arachidonic acids are vital to infants. I doubt that their importance disappears as we grow. Linoleic, an essential fatty acid, can't be synthesized by the body, and must be supplied in our food. Arachidonic, also essential, can be synthesized from available linoleic in the diet.

Because linoleic occurs in corn, cottonseed, peanut, safflower and soy oils, but not in olive or coconut oils, the former are preferred. Another problem with coconut for some is that its oil is saturated. As for olive oil, Barbara Apisson points out that, in cooking, olive oil burns very rapidly, losing food values. Olive oil fanciers do well to confine its use to salads and other noncooking uses.

Barbara's favorite mix for cookery—and I've adopted it—is safflower, sunflower and corn in equal proportions. Soy is nutritious but heavy for cookery.

Excellent F-sources are thin pie crusts or dainty cookies with sesame seeds, fresh soy meal, fresh ground nuts (not preroasted) and vegetables lightly cooked in unsaturated oils, not water—as well as the unsaturated oils themselves used in salads or general cookery.

Coronary patients of mine do well on these foods, along with homemade drink mixes containing lecithin and polyunsaturated oils of choice blenderized with grape concentrate (*petmez*) or a *little* maple syrup, possibly with a few ground nuts of choice, yeast powder, a dash of yogurt and pieces of raw zucchini. Experiment with combinations of these ingredients, omitting sweeteners if you prefer your homemade health cocktail straight—it's a boon to coronary patients and candidates.

VITAMIN K

Important in relation to prothrombin, vitamin K, as we have said, is a factor that causes normal blood clotting. Combined with C and rutin, vitamin K has been given by doctors to clear up stubborn nosebleeds. Those deficient in vitamin K, especially those with liver or gallbladder trouble, may need to be given injections of K by their doctors until the cause is cleared up.

The best vitamin-K sources are green leafy vegetables, botanicals, kelp, dulse, seaweed, salads, dill, parsley, oregano, mint leaves, alfalfa and lavender, added to soups, in drinks, all fresh as possible. Freshly chop or grind them and add them to meat loaf or fold them into gravies and sauces. Doesn't a window box or home garden make more sense as we go along?

Let's not glide over seaweed. Brown seaweed is a Japanese staple. In some places it provides up to a quarter of the day's diet. Norway, Sweden, Denmark, Iceland, Ireland and Scotland, to name just some seagirt lands, use seaweed as a prime culinary constituent.

Seaweed called porphyra, resembling spinach and tasting like oysters, is a Scottish favorite. The Irish relish crisp, tender leaves of sea lettuce or fresh dulse and use it dried in winter cooking. Health-food and gourmet shops here sell dried dulse. Seaweed called kelp—granules, powder or tablet—is getting popular here, too, served as salt (it contains 10 percent sea salt) and added to sauce, bread, soup, or sprinkled on potatoes, beans, lentils, bulgur, rice or salads. Research shows that kelp has a role in reducing the body's absorption of strontium 90.

Kelp and dulse are fine natural sources of vanadium, chromium, bromine, lithium and nearly all the trace elements bodies need, including some iodine and fluoride (see each of these in Chapter 5). Seaweed can also provide vitamins A, the B's, C, D and others, besides K.

Vegetarians should know about kelp and dulse, both sources of nutrients these people often lack because of aversion to meat and poultry. Other minerals in kelp are calcium, copper, boron, barium, strontium and zinc. *Warning:* Some barium, such as chloride, can be poisonous.

We get and need little vitamin K. An optimal diet can provide 2 mg. For normal people, that's enough. Pregnant women should be sure they're getting that much daily. Doctors may inject larger amounts before delivery to prevent hemorrhage by either mother or baby during birth; such injections also prevent a seriously K-deficient infant from suffering brain damage.

Vitamin K-influenced prothrombin is not the body's only clotting factor. A healthy liver, functioning digestive tract and unobstructed bile duct system, which most of us are born with, work together to extract all the needed vitamin K from our foods and store it in the liver for proper prothrombin regulation in the blood supply.

Malnutrition threatens this balance. Certain drugs do, too. Aspirin and salicylates in large doses, as well as quinine and quinidine, have been shown to suppress the liver's ability to form prothrombin. Sulfa drugs (sulfonamides) and other broad-spectrum antibiotics can also interfere with favorable bacteria in the intestines, reducing production of vitamin K. Other medications reported likely to slow clotting are thyroid drugs, such as dextrothyroxine and methyl or propyl thiouracil; certain anabolic steroids, which build up compounds in our metabolism; some radioactive compounds introduced into the body; and clofibrate, methyldopa and disulfiram.

Use of disulfiram, sometimes administered in cases of alcoholism, must always be monitored by a doctor, who will advise patients what symptoms this drug may cause. Another compound, levodopa, used in Parkinson's disease, may also produce internal bleeding, ulceration and anemia—symptoms arising from interference with vitamin-K (prothrombin) balance. Especially if there is liver disease, close contact between doctor and patient is necessary when these drugs are used.

Certain food-processing methods can lower vitamin-K content and allow bleeding. This is unhappily true of pasteurization in some cases. It is not true in unpasteurized milk. Chlorinated water, taken internally, also reduces the effectiveness of vitamin K. Where it is determined that bile mechanism is below par, people given K receive bile salts simultaneously. An alternative is an injection of vitamin K by the doctor. And since overdosing on K can be dangerous, nobody should mess around with it as a supplement without doctor's orders and supervision.

It's also been discovered that vitamin-A overdosing, especially where there is a low K intake, can cause vitamin-K deficiency. Vitamin K appears to work with vitamin E to prevent excessive clotting, but the reasons are unclear.

A Caucasus diet makes more and more sense as we discover how it produces in us naturally the nutrient combinations that keep our systems in balance. When we cite rat experiments, kindly dissenters often remind us that rats aren't people. But Caucasus centenarians *are* people.

In summary on vitamin K:

1. Those who don't and won't eat green vegetables, won't eat seaweed or such supplements as kelp, and those who habitually eat processed and overheated foods may be running the risk of vitamin-K deficiency.

2. While the need for vitamin K varies from person to person, those barely getting by on present diets may encounter sudden trouble if their livers act up, if they are exposed to bad cooking methods for the first time or if a number of special conditions develop, requiring drug therapy with the mentioned side effects.

Periodic onsets of diarrhea or colitis, or episodes of the flu or any infection requiring antibiotics while possibly depressing the appetite, are inevitable wasters of vitamin K. And remember that wide range of strange diets we complained about earlier and *their* inevitable interference with vitamin-K balance? Now estimate how many major clotting abnormalities figure in heart, vascular and other conditions mentioned. It should be clear that most causes of mortality involve blood clotting or the failure of blood to clot.

Since vitamin-K balance is merely a matter of proper nutrition for most of us, do you see now the absurdity of not eating green vegetables, snorting at seaweed and ignoring other sources of this vital nutrient? And doesn't the massive number of deaths relating to clotting and nonclotting suggest how *attention to this one aspect of nutrition all by itself* can make a big difference in potential candidates for the age of 100?

VITAMIN P

Vitamin P (for permeability) will get us arguments. But existing research convinces me that (1) there *is* such a thing as vitamin P, (2) it works somewhat as vitamin C does, and (3) it works with vitamin C to prevent scurvy and counteract artery disease, capillary leakage, fragility of our smallest blood vessels, bleeding tendencies and high blood pressure.

I have engaged in this research myself and have followed the work of others. We used guinea pigs and humans, testing with pure ascorbic acid—that is, we used natural vitamin C in our extracts. Then we compared what happened to our subjects when we added rutin, extract of walnut drupe (an excellent source of vitamins C and P) and finally the whole package: C, the P complex, K, the B complex, and minerals, including calcium—in sum, all the vitamins and minerals known to be connected with clotting. We observed that the system works best when all these favorably influencing food factors are included in the diet.

Drugs and synthetics are available for coagulation. Still others are available for the opposite effect—to inhibit clotting in phlebitis and other conditions. But these do not always work. Heparin, dicoumarol, plasmin—they are all imperfect performers. Plasmin works only when given early. Even K injections can come too late for specific situations, such as brain injury, bleeding ulcer and general gastrointestinal bleeding.

We naturally conclude that prevention is better than cure, particularly prevention through everyday diet. P-complex sources are rutin, hesperidin, citrin, citrus bioflavonoid and bioflavonoid. You find them as additives to some but not all multipurpose vitamin tablets.

Doubt is often expressed as to whether these substances really do us any good. It's true that storage of the product can present problems. Undue exposure to light, heat, lack of freshness of product and a spate of similar variables exercise oxidizing influences on the P complex just as in other nutrients I've mentioned.

Our government doesn't think much of bioflavonoids. Such pills are labelled, by requirement, "Need in human nutrition not determined." But government opinion notwithstanding, I am too familiar with the fact that serious clotting or bleeding cases continue defying doctors and that the smartest thing any individual can do in such circumstances is try to prevent the condition from developing by making a serious effort to eat right.

Those healthy original and succeeding generations of Caucasians have been getting plenty of vitamin P, particularly from *fresh* lettuce, such as I wish were more available here; from their currants, cherries, berries, rose hips, apricots, apples, grapes, tomatoes, potatoes, carrots, parsnips, turnips (greens included) and peas; *and* from their wintertime fruits, such as prunes, raisins, dried apricots and peppers (green, red and red-green).

If you trust your rutin/bioflavonoid source, if you have assurance of high standards in handling reliably healthy sources and freshness, you may prefer taking vitamin P as a supplement to relying on drugs after either bleeding or clotting problems appear. I take rutin. I have bioflavonoids in the all-purpose vitamins I use as supplements. I believe we all need these.

VITAMIN Q

Professor Arnold J. Quick of Wisconsin University, first known for his discovery of dicoumarol, isolated vitamin Q, an anticoagulant factor. Vitamin Q is different from E, which tests have shown to have anticoagulant factors, too. Vitamin Q appears in the greater legume group, such as clover, alfalfa, soy. A notable quality of vitamin Q taken as food is that it cannot harm us, as anti-clotting drugs can (see vitamin P).

Vitamin Q negates the harmful effects of clotting. Where bits of clots break off in the leg, the brain and in the heart, as in coronary occlusion, vitamin Q works against their blocking vessels wherever they might tend to pile up, damming blood flow with dangerous to disastrous results. Vitamin Q, consumed as food, goes no further. Drugs may or may not know where to stop after doing the same job.

American doctors take little stock in vitamin E's anticoagulant properties. But vitamin-E advocates report "luck" in preventing subsequent blood-clotting when used after one or more incidents have already taken place. Even so, most doctors oppose the idea that anything dietary, except omission of sodium, helps treat or prevent heart disease.

A few of us have obtained good results from vitamins E, C and the C complex (see vitamin P), as well as B_6 in the mix. More research is needed on vitamin Q. But my conviction is that the nutrient group of which it is part is beneficial in some serious conditions too prevalent in our times. Proof will come along.

VITAMIN U

Ever hear of it? It's the vitamin scientists are still trying to find. It's so rapidly destroyed that no way has yet been found to preserve it.

Vitamin U was named by Dr. Garnett Cheney as a component in fresh natural foods, one that exerts healing action on peptic ulcers caused by lack of fresh foods. He reached his conclusions after treating soldiers who came down with peptic ulcers on K-ration diets. Compared with those on regular army food, a high percentage of K-ration consumers had ulcers. Since K rations, like fresh foods, provided ascorbic acid, Dr. Cheney decided that, in these cases, "some other vitamin factor found in fresh foods and ordinary service diets must be missing."

Although vitamin U has yet to be isolated, extracts of foods can be shown to contain this something-of-value not found in K rations. My husband, Kegan, and I got involved in the quest for vitamin U. We were experiencing success against ulcers with some of our extracts. Other scientists worked with us. We concentrated on wound healing and treatment of ulceration in animals.

The information on fresh cabbage extract, on which Dr. Cheney based his observations, frustrated us. It's been established that vitamin U is different from C, the B complex and other vitamins we know better. But its proneness to destruction has kept vitamin U from our grasp.

Heating, aging and storage all destroy it. Fresh and raw, foods rich in vitamin U are celery, cereal grasses, fresh greens, types of cabbage, raw egg yolks, unpasteurized fresh milk (animals that forage appear to get it from range herbs and grasses), and certain vegetables and freshly extracted animal fats.

Is vitamin U real? Ulcers treated with vitamin-U rich extracts heal three to six times faster than those treated by conventional bland diets with milk and alkalis. That's in seven to ten days instead of thirty-seven to forty-two. So vitamin U is real enough. One day we'll isolate it and use it more reliably than we do now.

That brings us to the end of our list of vitamins until someone discovers another which may qualify as V. But you're still urged to read carefully as we go through the list of minerals in Chapter 5.

5. Nutrients We Must Have: Minerals

In this chapter I want you to meet the elements of good nutrition. Do you remember our introductory description of the body as a fountain of youth? In addition to vitamins, we need minerals and chemicals in that fountain to keep it youthful longer years. There's quite a list of them. Some are needed in minute amounts, literally traces; others are essential in larger quantities. We don't have either exact or final data on minerals any more than we do on vitamins, but the gaps are filling all the time. My younger readers are going to live to see many more of them filled as researchers develop new knowledge about how to use nature's yields to help them remain healthy longer.

I'm going to list alphabetically the minerals I think you should know best. What you're about to see is by no means the entire list. It includes trace elements we appear to need.

BROMINE

Commercially, bromine is used in antiknock gasoline and other nonnutritive ways. A natural element characterized by its deep red color and caustic, foul-smelling vapor, only a small amount of bromide salt is necessary to humans for normal liver function, proper brain performance and the operation of the adrenal, thyroid and pituitary glands.

There are bromide traces in our blood and nails. Bromine deficiency has been associated with mental abnormalities. Bromine, chlorine, fluorine and iodine are four halogens important to health.

There's no RDA for bromine, but it's part of our makeup. I would say a trace belongs in our diet. Traces can be found in edible animal glands, mussels, kelp, sea plants, seawater and elsewhere in nature.

CALCIUM

We are "doing" minerals alphabetically but can't bring up calcium without referring to vitamin D and phosphorus. You'll see why in a moment. First, you may know calcium is the major mineral for growth and maintenance of bones and teeth, but it has other important uses in the body. For instance, proper calcium supply and metabolism are essential to prevention of muscle cramps and spasms, which are usually also related to vitamin-D deficiency.

Calcium is best absorbed by the body when there is enough vitamin D and phosphorus in our diet. It's agreed we need some 800 mg. of calcium daily. I believe it should be more on the order of 2,200 mg. daily, together with adequate supplies of vitamin D and phosphorus (see separate headings). Calcium supply figures in bone formation and bone cellular replacement, as well as in normal blood clotting, pulse rate, muscle tone, heart contractions and nervous-system balance.

Get as much calcium as possible from the natural sources listed below. However, a modest daily supplement is 1,000 mg. (1 gram). The elderly probably need supplements of 1 to 2 grams (g.) a day. In osteoporosis ("softening" of the bones), doctors commonly suggest daily supplements of 3 g.

Osteoporosis is all too common among the elderly (it is also found in malnourished children). As people get older, bone-substance breakdown often accelerates, a factor that makes old people quite literally shrink. Where calcium deficiency does exist, vulnerability to osteoporosis is high and broken bones often result. Weak skeletal structures in children produce the same problem.

Such conditions can be stopped by increasing calcium/phosphorus intake. Where older people take less milk in their diets, they should be taking more.

Whole milk is our biggest natural calcium source. Cheeses come second. Other sources are salmon canned with the bones (which should be eaten), other fish, meat, eggs, turnip greens, mustard greens, breads and cereals, legumes and nuts. Yogurt, buttermilk, seaweed, kelp, carob flour, defatted soybean flour, and sesame seeds are also good sources of calcium.

If you hate milk and cheese or are allergic to them, supplementation is important. Otherwise calcium deficiency is a major risk.

Even when you take enough calcium, it could pass through you unused. Not enough acid in your duodenum, causing excess alkalinity, can react against absorption of calcium. Oxalic acid, found in spinach, chard, rhubarb, cocoa and beet greens, reduces normal calcium availability. That argues against using milk or cheese in the same meal with any of these foods.

Protein and hormones are two other important factors in healthy bones. Both children and the elderly can be borderline protein eaters. It is possible for a child with adequate natural enzymes, adequate calcium, phosphorus and vitamin-D intake to have bone problems due to low or borderline protein intake.

Some calcium supplements give you more available calcium than others. Tests show that calcium from oyster shells is more readily available than from any other known source, which leads me to write again, read your labels.

Some medications cause calcium problems. Research indicates that tranquilizers, phenobarbitol, muscle relaxants, anticonvulsants or oral prescriptions for diabetes attack vitamin D and, by so doing, reduce calcium's effectiveness in the diet. Obviously, something as fundamental to health as calcium requires your serious attention—as do quantities of whole milk plus supplementation.

CHLORINE

The recommended daily intake of chlorine (as chloride) for healthy persons is .5 g. Sodium chloride is important for blood stability and the work of other body fluids. It's important in cell composition and cell function. And as you may know, hydro*chloric* acid is necessary to digestion.

A number of sodium-salt compounds are needed for normal heart activity and for regulating both acid-alkali balance and osmotic pressure (absorption of blood and body fluids between tissues). Dramatic deficiency is found in some cases of vomiting, diarrhea, dysentery, sprue, cholera or colitis. When such conditions are prolonged, excessive body-salt loss can be accompanied by dehydration if the losses aren't restored quickly.

Hospitals treat these cases as they do shock and burn victims—with saline solutions. Intravenous feedings often play a lifesaving role.

Chlorine gas is poisonous, highly irritating and potentially fatal. Chlorine can also nullify vitamin E. People drinking heavily chlorinated water should change their water source if for no other reason than recent reports of carcinogens appearing in chlorinated river waters. Our Berkeley water, during our vitamin E studies, proved to be heavily chlorinated. We had to take precautions not just for our rats but also for ourselves.

Vitamins E and A, calcium, phosphorus and good protein balance in your diet will, by overcoming induced losses, protect your heart, muscles and sexual performance.

CHROMIUM

This substance is not just for the shiny parts of your car. Though no RDA has been set for chromium, we probably need about 2 mg. daily. I believe chromium is a vital body mineral, a youth mineral.

In the Caucasus, I found the soil exceptionally rich in chromium. Volcanic upheavals and floods deposited a wealth of chromium, copper, zinc, molybdenum, iron and aluminum in Noah's Ark country, naturally enriching its breadbasket and grazing grounds.

Armenians reap harvests of mineral-rich foods from soils containing dolomite (magnesium, calcium), diatomite (shell, fishbone, tooth remnants, calcified remains of microscopic sea life), rock salts, phosphorite, high-grade clays, marble as crystallized limestone and deposits of silver and gold. (Remember their sheep with the gold-plated teeth?) Copper, cobalt, uranium ores and still other mineral riches are also compacted into Armenia's soil strata.

Where do we obtain chromium? In cocoa, cloves, unrefined botanical herbs, other spices, grape molasses, the residue of molasses or dark sugar and unrefined whole grains, to name the sources I've used myself. It's also found in traces in tree or fruit sugars, shellfish, chicken and some fresh-cooked meats.

Dr. Henry A. Schroeder of Dartmouth Medical School's Trace Minerals Laboratory, with whom I maintain contact, and Dr. Walter Mertz have labelled chromium foods keys to youthful blood vessels. From my own practice and research, I know that wheat, botanicals, vitamins C and E and other natural antioxidants such as are in whole seeds, grains, drupes, fruits, green nuts—with gel or bulk fiber added—are a chromium youth cocktail of high value when taken together or in such combinations as may be available.

I hear from Dr. Schroeder that no supplemental tablet we can buy today is as beneficial as chromium from natural sources. Be guided accordingly.

In cane sugar-growing areas of the world, crude fiber residues of sugar factories have long been prized as a food source. The Middle Easterners and Orientals know this and import the residue, which is rich in chromium. I learned from a Japanese doctor that his countrymen bake this food leftover with beans, adding its mineral-rich values to their diets. They also add it to whole-grain puddings. (See *anoushabour* in our recipe section, a Caucasus favorite.) This crude fiber is also seen in a spread for whole-grain breads.

It's a sardonic fact that the leftovers of sugar manufacture are so beneficial to those who eat it, while the prime product, refined white sugar, bestows great dangers on the civilizations that are addicted to it. For when we swallow white sugar as candy, sweetened drinks, sugared sweets or pastries on an empty stomach, *any chromium we may have taken into our tissues is wasted.* A cruel paradox this!

Clove and cinnamon teas contain chromium. So does cocoa—but not chocolate, which we adore so here. When rums, dried fruit, citrus, vine-ripened grapes, honey and other tree syrups originate in chromium-rich soil, there's chromium in all of them. *Petmez* has it, too.

Animals that graze on the natural yield of rich Caucasus soils pass along chromium in their livers, hearts, lungs, spleens and kidneys. Other chromium sources are eggs, butter, roe, caviar, some unrefined vegetable oils, brans, coarse-grain residues from flour mills and some of our water. Commercial animal feed can provide enough chromium, if eaten, to save a human life.

Where there's any threat to chromium nutrition, people should strictly avoid refined white sugar and white flour, chromium-poor starches and such saturated fats as margarine and hydrogenates. They should strictly avoid just about all commercially prepared baked goods, juices and beverages. And they should keep away from commercial jellies, candies, sweet cakes, tarts, crackers, cookies, colas, sodas, sauces, cake and pudding mixes *and anything else loaded with refined white sugar, commercial glucose or starch, white flour or other refined-grain products.*

Dr. Schroeder has become convinced through his work that the American habit of eating such foods gives us 60 percent of our calories from them in a diet that not only does not provide enough chromium for our needs, but one that robs us of chromium reserves we're born with by failing to replace our urinary losses.

He sees our prevailing fondness for chromium-poor foods depriving our systems of the chromium needed for the metabolism of our excesses in junk foods. The result, he has concluded, is a disease very common today, attacking the arteries (atherosclerosis) by gradually hardening buildups, deposits of cholesterol and other fatty substances, which narrow the arteries at points where they become roadblocks to blood clots, crippling or killing their victims.

In research which Dr. Schroeder cites, the draining of chromium from the body was shown to produce elevated cholesterol levels, abnormal sugar tolerance, heart and vascular derangements, diabetes, strokes, hemorrhages, hardening of the arteries, coronary diseases—and premature aging and death.

We are born with adequate chromium. By their late teens, Americans show chromium deficiency. Tissue analysis in Japan and the Caucasus shows four times as much chromium at the same ages. This difference continues to be observable into old age. Our dietary habits are making us fall behind, something that I am convinced is costing us dearly in survival and longevity.

In this book, we are searching for healthier, longer life. Solid, credible research, such as Dr. Schroeder's, has indicated that chromium, zinc and the antioxidant vitamins C and E, in an optimal diet which includes certain botanicals, supply basic youth factors vital to better health and longer life.

Science doesn't create such a truth. Scientists, searching for all their professional lives, if funded enough, smart enough and maybe lucky enough, can *confirm* such a truth and perhaps begin to explain it.

In the Caucasus I saw a neat balance between tradition and progress—an instinctive marriage between what time has proved valuable in nutrition and what modern man learned about sanitation, preparation and processing before commerce and industry corrupted that learning for profit.

Historians, not doctors, may better say one day why and how a kind of instinctive native shrewdness led Caucasus peoples to "bring up" their soils, reclaim nature's best from nature and live longer, healthier lives as a result.

With our resources and their natural diet, we can turn from a citizenry dying prematurely to a people who make an all-out effort to upgrade our diets, lengthen our lives and make living what it was supposed to be.

I never see our mission more clearly than when I think of chromium imbalance and its role in shortening life.

COPPER

Copper is classified as a trace element. We need only 2 mg. a day in our diet, *but that much is essential,* because copper must be present in the blood for conversion of iron into hemoglobin. As Wintrobe and Cartright, Hopkins colleagues, concluded in a fine paper on the subject, copper, little as we need, is vital to the formation of healthy blood. Its lack can be a factor in anemia.

Copper also relates to pigment formation by making an amino acid (via the enzyme tyrosinase) usable, and it helps the body utilize its supply of vitamin C, playing a role in vitamin-C metabolism.

The easiest thing to remember about copper is that it is important to our red blood cells, the oxygen carriers in our bloodstreams. The mineral works best when present with chromium, iodine, cobalt and zinc. In combination, these strengthen formation of red blood cells and contribute effectively to good health.

Safe natural sources of copper are: almonds, egg yolks, whole wheat, molasses, some fruits (plums, prunes, apricots, black mission figs, loganberries), some vegetables (peas, beans, lentils) and liver. Copper is also found in seafood (shrimps, clams and oysters).

Speaking of the benefits of taking minerals in combinations, let's see how well Caucasus favorites stand up in this regard. Bulgur combines iron, copper, cobalt and vitamin E with other nutrients. Liver and other organs contain copper, iron, cobalt, zinc, B-complex, vitamin A and other nutrients. Add onion and dulse for iodine. Add garlic for vitamin C, sulfide and the nutrients that were covered earlier. The Caucasian habit of mixing foods has been one of their greatest health aids.

FLUORINE/FLUORIDE

Fluorine is a powerful element of the chlorine family, in one form useful in etching glass. It's so strong that it is difficult to store safely. The body needs it, too, as the salt fluoride. By now, so many years into the argument, almost everyone has an opinion on fluoridation of water to improve the teeth.

In places where small quantities of the mineral occur naturally in water, some of the healthiest teeth known are found in the inhabitants. But add just a little more fluoride and mottling plus some of the *worst* tooth conditions known are observed. Adding fluoride to water supply, highly controversial, remains open to serious questions.

We do appear to need about 500 mcg. (micrograms) of fluoride in our diet although there's no RDA here, either. The mineral is a small component in bones and teeth. There is medical evidence that too much can be just as harmful as too little

My not wading into the fluoride-in-water controversy will disappoint those on either side. But I can't contribute to the fluoride furor when nothing I read on either side stands up to objective criteria.

Fluoride is found in our nails, blood, skin and hair chiefly, but no data yet compiled enables me to say to you how important this mineral, as a factor in diet, might be to us. We find it in tea, artificially and naturally fluoridated waters, bone meal, whole-fish meal and sea plants.

IODINE

There is no question about iodine—we need from .15 to .3 mg. a day. A supplement of .1 to .2 mg. a day might be a good idea. Don't get it from any bottle, marked poison, intended to keep minor cuts from infecting.

Iodine is an essential nutrient of the thyroid-hormonal system. If there isn't enough present in the thyroid gland, the pituitary gland contributes a hormone that stimulates the thyroid to enlarge. This enlargement is the condition called goiter, probably entirely preventable with normal iodine intake.

A normal thyroid regulates the body metabolism working in harmony with the endocrine-gland system. Thyroid hormones must be present for adequate human growth. Also, iodine aids in the oxidation of proteins and fats and stimulates the circulatory system.

In Japan, where iodine-rich seaweed is a staple of diet, there is less goiter than anywhere else in the world. Other foods from the sea contain iodine, but I suggest supplementation because, unless you eat seafood regularly (you should) and seaweed regularly (you should), the amount of iodine you get every day depends on how rich or poor in iodine your soil is. That can't be reliably measured with food coming from almost anywhere these days.

Deliberate use of iodized salt in areas (such as Michigan) known for high incidence of goiter provided such excellent results in reducing goiter incidence that all of us should intelligently consider buying iodized salt, now generally available, as a substitute for ordinary table salt. Certainly, in goiter-prone families, this is a simple and obvious remedy, probably already suggested by doctors.

IRON

Normally we need 10 to 12 mg. of iron a day. The government recommends 18 mg. daily for pregnant and lactating women. In cases of bleeding (for instance, menstruation) or diarrhea, the body needs extra iron. Supplementation is important in such conditions and, to prevent deficiency, it is a good idea for most of us.

We normally consume 1 mg. of iron a day. The rest of what's in us is, by and large, broken down and re-used. The difference between the 1 mg. per day we expend and what we need as a supplement—as I indicated, 10 to 12 mg.—is insurance against deficiency.

Why is this? We do not absorb all the iron we ingest. Also, U.S. surveys show that one diet in five doesn't have enough iron to start with. So, where do you get iron? From some enriched breakfast cereal or from some enriched white bread? Probably. Yes, there's iron in those enriched junk foods, but they do more harm to us than good. So, iron-wise, and otherwise, it's safer to turn to whole natural foods.

The relationship between iron and vitamin C, a very complicated matter, is lately getting increased scientific study. You must have sufficient vitamin C for absorption of iron. But one person in five is conceded to be deficient in vitamin C. Some of us think the number is higher. The one-in-five ratio means that 43 million Americans are defective in iron absorption because they are deficient in vitamin C. Still more millions are iron-deficient because their food comes from deficient soils or for other reasons.

Iron deficiency shows up in other circumstances. Recent anemia studies measuring vitamin B_{12} in human blood serum show that 1 g. a day of vitamin C given to paraplegics at the Bronx Veterans Administration Hospital was related to their low B_{12} levels. Vitamin C had been given to balance the effects of long-term antibiotic dosage. According to normal criteria, the patients were receiving enough B_{12}, but the gram a day of vitamin C somehow blocked the body's ability to use the B_{12}.

The same patients were then given large doses of B_{12}, with and without vitamin C. The results confirmed that, when high amounts of C are taken, the way many pill-popping Americans take them these days, excessive ascorbic acid destroys up to 95 percent of the B_{12} content of the diet.

How does this relate to iron? Interestingly, if the liver gets enough iron from meals or supplements or both, iron in the liver or bile will prevent much B_{12} destruction from excessive vitamin C. *But,* scientists report, *too much* iron in the system, instead of protecting B_{12} from destruction from excessive vitamin C, will lend a hand in destroying B_{12}. You'll be glad to read that the amount of vitamin C we recommend as a supplement, particularly in time-release form, does not destroy B_{12}.

When we see the alarming way nutrients can cancel each other out, there's something downright appealing in a whole food diet imitating the people of the Caucasus, where nature has been a kind chemist.

LITHIUM

The lightest known metal, lithium, is used commercially in metallurgy and nuclear technology and is common in such work as potter's glazing. We get a form of lithium in our diet, about 2 mg. a day, but it is classified as a nonessential trace element in human nutrition. (So are a dozen or so more I won't go into.)

I would skip lithium except for the fact that this mineral, found in the ocean and in rock formations, has been identified with successful treatment of depression and reduction of physical damage from alcoholism by cutting down drinking bouts.

Lithium overdosing is dangerous. Its level in the blood requires careful monitoring. Lithium, used as a salt substitute, has caused imbalance in body fluids and death by replacing sodium in tissue. Lithium may be a subject to discuss with your doctor in cases of severe depression or alcoholism.

Sea-influenced soils probably add traces to our diet. What we get in our food seems to provide our needs, far from perfectly understood.

MAGNESIUM

People who get a lot of calcium in their diets are apt to absorb less magnesium. Calcium and magnesium battle one another to get into our systems. This and many other factors have led specialists to the conclusion that there's a great deal of magnesium deficiency in this land of junk food. Some books claim that the whole nation is magnesium-deficient. Discount that by any percentage you like and it is still quite an indictment!

Daily need for magnesium is 300-350 mg., possibly a little more. As we said, magnesium must be present for vitamin B_6 to be utilized by the body. Supplement with 50-100 mg. daily.

The best sources of magnesium are almonds, Brazil nuts, peanuts and peanut flour, cottonseed flour, defatted soybean flour, soybeans, wheat bran, wheat germ and brewer's yeast. Most nuts and seeds contain varying amounts. It's also found in barley, beet greens, fresh corn, millet, whole grains, oats, sesame seeds, dried whey—and there's some in apricots, raw asparagus, bananas, lima beans, beets, chard, dandelion greens, lentils, blackstrap molasses, peas, brown rice and rye flour.

If there's so much in so many places, you may ask, how can anyone say we are deficient, or worse still that we are *all* deficient in magnesium? It used to be thought none of us *could* be. Maybe our eating habits have changed. Too, lots of people suspect quackery in whole natural foods. Some people reason that even if the entire food industry pours refined white sugar and flour and convenience food additives into us, anyone who calls an entire industry wrong must be some kind of nut. Because people reason that way, it's possible to be shortchanged on magnesium.

We need magnesium throughout our bodies. Most goes into our bones, but it's needed in our blood, soft tissues and cells. And since a calcium-rich diet (lots of milk and cheese) makes it hard for magnesium to be absorbed, we'd better all see that we get the minimum supplement in addition to a diet of magnesium foods to insure an average adult intake of 300-350 mg., as recommended above.

Is magnesium deficiency fact or fantasy? Judge for yourself. More housewives than we can count suffer from that tired-all-over feeling that won't go away—the blahs. When doctors suspect magnesium deficiency, a confirming blood test is followed by almost certain cure. I've cleared up foggy memories and taken away countless blahs with a high-magnesium diet and supplements.

Magnesium is also important to enzyme utility and in energy metabolism. Its lack is seen in alcoholism. Since magnesium is needed throughout our tissues and cells, chronic deficiency can lead to destruction of our tiny capillaries. In the brain, this is very serious.

Magnesium is important, too, for muscle contraction. The heart is a muscle! Quite definitely, add magnesium to minerals important for you.

MANGANESE

Here is still another key body-building metallic element. The body seems to need 15 to 25 mg. daily to utilize thiamine (vitamin B_1) and choline (B complex). You've read how important they are. Manganese, which enables them to work, is equally important. This mineral is also vital in carbohydrate metabolism and urea formation.

An average "intelligent" diet should give you all you need,

especially if you know that blueberries, buckwheat, wheat bran, legumes and nuts are its richest natural sources. If you take an all-purpose vitamin/mineral supplement (and I hope you do), look for a modest amount of manganese in it.

MOLYBDENUM

We don't get or need much molybdenum. About 100 mcg. has been estimated to be our daily need. Too much molybdenum is not good for us. It has been recognized that we should get some in our diet, but until fairly recently it was supposed that we didn't need it very much. Now there's interest in the possible role of excess molybdenum in certain forms of cancer. In this connection it has been observed that a high-protein diet is instrumental in keeping the body free of molybdenum buildup.

Soybeans and other legumes, leafy vegetables, liver, kidney and whole-grain cereals provide natural molybdenum. There's some in yeast, too, and other organ meats.

Molybdenum is necessary to the functioning of some enzymes and may be important in extracting energy from fats. If it's shown as a trace in supplements, it isn't harmful. But, at most, we need very little.

NICKEL

Nobody has figured out how much nickel we need. But in common with our atmosphere and the earth's crust, a minute amount of nickel is part of us. Authorities believe nickel is necessary for hormonal and glandular activity, especially for proper function of the thyroid and adrenals. Intakes far above the body's need can lead to trouble, but few are likely to be overexposed unless inhaling nickel dust at work.

There is little nickel in animal foods. What we get comes largely from whole grains and cereals, herring, oysters, ordinary tea and buckwheat seeds.

Suspicion is growing among food chemists that nickel is more important than we know and that, in a generally deficient diet, nickel deficiency probably contributes to poor health as part of that picture. Obviously, further study is needed to tell us more about nickel's role in human nutrition.

PHOSPHORUS

Most of what I wanted to tell you about phosphorus is its connection with calcium (see calcium). Nutritionists say we need about 1½ times more phosphorus than we do calcium. If we need 2,200 mgs. of calcium, somewhere around 3,000 mg. (3 g.) of phosphorus should do us very nicely. That's not a lot. The body stores excess calcium/phosphorus as reserves. You are far better off with those reserves than with just enough. A sudden calcium/phosphorus need with no reserves to draw on robs the bones of replacement and maintenance nutrients leading to conditions discussed earlier under calcium.

Get plenty of phosphorus in food and look for more in your all-purpose supplement. A gram or more won't harm you a bit. Foods rich in phosphorus are pumpkin seeds (among the richest sources), rice bran, wheat bran, wheat germ and rice polishings; sesame, sunflower and safflower seeds; brewer's yeast, soybeans, defatted soybean flour and sunflower-seed flour; kidney beans, peanuts, almonds, filberts; and flounder, chicken and liver. Yogurt, cheeses and milk also provide rich amounts of phosphorus along with good quantities of calcium.

POTASSIUM

We need 3,000 mg. (3 g.) daily of this alkali metal element (taken as the salt) for proper muscle contraction, normal nerve function and normal flow of messages between the brain and the body's action stations.

Potassium supports formation of storage depots of glycogen (how we form and store fats and proteins). Potassium operates largely in the fluid medium of our cells, where it regulates fluid balances.

When people fill up with fluid, as women do premenstrually or as people do from overeating salty foods, or as happens in some heart and kidney disorders, doctors often prescribe diuretics to make them urinate frequently. What departs from the body is largely saline solution plus potassium. Frequently doctors will prescribe effervescent potassium with diuretics or will suggest oranges, grapefruit, bananas or other fruits high in potassium.

Meats, grains, legumes and vegetables are good potassium sources. Cucumbers and parsnips are especially good.

Warning: Do not buy potassium pills on your own. Fatal ulcers of the small intestines have been caused by pill-form potassium. The effervescent tablet, diluted in water, overcomes this problem. Supplement under your doctor's guidance.

SELENIUM

Here's another trace mineral we don't know enough about. Experiments show that it can both inhibit and cause cancer—just the kind of information that makes it difficult to talk about selenium at all. But I do have *some* information and some feelings about this mineral.

We don't know how much we need. But people get it naturally in meats, especially organ meats; whole-grain cereals, nuts, milk products, vegetables and fruit. If you are taking a good all-purpose vitamin/mineral supplement, there's probably selenium in it.

Animal experiments have proved that vitamin E and selenium in combination are important to one another's function in chickens and in other nonhuman species. In 1973, the Food and Drug Administration (FDA) recognized this fact by allowing the addition of selenium in small quantities to some animal feeds. This was, the FDA said, to promote better growth while fighting disease and costly deaths of livestock. The amount approved is small enough to prevent selenium buildup in tissues that could be passed on to humans.

Experiments show that vitamin E in animal diets helps destroy harmful effects of fatty substances in the blood. If vitamin E is not present, selenium appears to do the job. If neither is present, there is sure trouble for the animal.

While we have no data yet on experiments with humans, prudent people will conclude, as I have, that the selenium present in whole foods with other high-nutrient values is a good thing—and that animal tests showing a supportive relationship between vitamin E and selenium are one more reason to take vitamin E seriously.

SILICON

The establishment says, not unanimously, that there is no real proof that silicon does us any good. It has been shown important in plant life—there's a lot of it around. Some authorities, and I agree with them, impressed with the fact that there is silicon in our tooth enamel; nerve, muscle and connective tissue; blood; skin; nails and hair believe we require some 3 mg. daily to support all this activity, whether its value has been proved or not.

Health faddists say silicon is important to disease resistance. I find no proof that this is true. Astrologers advise Leos (late July into August) to eat foods rich in silicon. These are buckwheat products, mushrooms, raw carrots, whole tomatoes (stem and all), seedy figs, wild strawberries with grit in them, savoy cabbage and pages more.

When someone proves silicon is important to us—and someone will—I'll be glad to know it. Meantime, I doubt that we need supplements to replace what we use if we are eating a normal diet.

SODIUM

The RDA on sodium varies with the authors making recommendations. My best guess is we need about 4,500 mg. a day under normal circumstances. In normal dietary choices, we get that much.

Even those on salt-free diets need some sodium for health and survival. Why? It aids in the formation of digestive juices. It is everywhere inside us. Its regulatory function is much like that of chloride. It helps regulate the acid-base balance of the body and osmotic pressures. It is plainly of major importance.

But it is a mixed blessing. Blood cells, measured as hematocrit, comprise some 40 percent of the blood. They are composed almost entirely of potassium and contain virtually no sodium. The other 60 percent fraction of the blood contains important amounts of sodium. And as we may all know, excessive sodium in our systems causes the body to retain fluids, sometimes to our peril.

Skin, urine and stool escape valves provide relief from excessive sodium in normal people. But people with heart and artery diseases must eliminate as much salt from their diets as possible.

To put the problem simply: Salt is vital to healthy people and can be dangerous to sick people.

SULFUR

I have concluded that we require about .8 to .9 g. of sulfur daily, which is largely available in protein foods. It is a constituent of the protein makeup of every cell in the body. If your diet is adequate in quality protein, you're getting enough sulfur.

That's important because sulfur works with a number of amino acids and with insulin, heparin, thiamine and biotin, among other items, to keep us healthy.

Sulfur has been part of our earth's composition since the beginning of time. It would be unnatural if, in its pervasive presence, we didn't require it for normal functioning.

VANADIUM

A trace of vanadium is vital, but nobody's sure how much is needed. Yet vanadium deficiency leads to teeth, bone and liver-cholesterol-fat metabolism abnormalities.

Vanadium does pose a deficiency problem. It is not added back when food processing destroys it. There is apparent need for vanadium to be added to animal feeds and fertilizers so that more of it can get into human consumption. Little as we need, evidence is mounting that many of us aren't getting that much from U.S. vegetables or meat.

Vanadium should be available in gelatin or bone meal. But domestic animals that supply our gelatin and bone meal are themselves deficient in this element. For supplementation, we should buy bone meal from areas of nondepletion. Gelatin and bone meal from South American countries (I'm surest of Argentina) should contain vanadium. Adding this gelatin and/or bone meal to what you eat may help lower cholesterol levels.

Excessive amounts of vanadium are not as harmful as excessive doses of other minerals. Because there's vanadium in petroleum products, petroleum waste workers have been found with green tongues that returned to normal color when workers left their jobs.

Vanadium is also found in dulse, kelp and all other types of seaweed. By taking those products for their other qualities, you'll get a vanadium plus, too.

Reports show vanadium can be inhaled from the air, is in the seas around us and in soils in certain areas. We need to know more about vanadium than we do. We know now that vanadium has a role in cholesterol levels. People who work with vanadium show lower cholesterol levels than the rest of us. By contrast, tests show that low vanadium levels go with elevated cholesterol counts. Eating vanadium-rich gelatin lowers the cholesterol count on examination.

Plainly, vanadium is another mineral important for healthy years.

ZINC

In 1974, zinc received the official government RDA of 15 mg. for average adults. It was about time.

Older men are prone to prostate trouble caused or aggravated by zinc deficiency. They are well-advised to get even more zinc than the RDA. Pregnant women are allowed 20 mg. daily, lactating females 25 mg. A good supplement for older men, if not both sexes in later life, is 20 to 25 mg.

There is growing evidence that the refining and processing of foods robs us of zinc, too. The government requires fortification to make up for losses in iron, but nobody has lobbied hard enough yet for zinc, vanadium and other trace minerals. It will come.

What about zinc supplements for better sexual performance? You decide. Next only to the muscle coating of the eye, the greatest zinc concentration in the body is found in the male prostate gland, with high concentration in the sperm, too. Conservatives may argue that these concentrations don't necessarily imply a role in sexual performance. I can't believe there is no relationship. A prudent person, if he's interested in sexual performance (and other reports that link zinc deficiency to a spectrum of human ailments), would be very much interested in zinc supplementation.

Zinc deficiency also seems to go hand in hand with inability, in certain mental illnesses, to dispose of copper normally. And there is growing evidence that an oversupply of copper causing depression can be reduced by a zinc-manganese attack, combined with high doses of vitamin C. Remember, copper kills vitamin C. If tests show high copper concentration associated with mental problems, there is reason to consider with your doctor a megavitamin approach emphasizing vitamin C, zinc and manganese.

Some other zinc-related factors: 1) Lead and cadmium, released in traffic pollution, attack available zinc and can cause trouble. 2) Loss of taste appears associated with low zinc levels. 3) Tests show zinc supplementation can reverse aging signs in human hair and acne in human skin. 4) Zinc ointments have helped cure wounds for years. 5) Low zinc levels appear in hardening of the arteries. Cases treated with zinc have shown marked improvement. 6) Low zinc levels have been associated with cirrhosis of the liver and with lung cancer. 7) Zinc plays an interesting role in relation to the scarce B vitamin, folic acid. Low zinc levels in animals have been found where folic acid was low. Something of the same relationship exists between zinc and vitamin A. How much vitamin A is available for the body's use seems to depend on how much zinc we store. Again, we have evidence that efficient nutrient availability is interlinked—we need them all to get the full benefit of each.

Fish and shellfish are our best zinc sources, most notably herring, oysters and clams. Unprocessed whole-grain cereals are also good zinc sources. There is some in whole wheat, brewer's yeast, rice, liver and beef, peas, corn, egg yolks, carrots and milk.

We see again and again how America's romance with processed foods, refined white-sugar and white-flour foods costs us dearly in lost nutrients. Zinc has the distinction of being at the end of an alphabet of items of which this is true.

I have listed here only the minerals that I feel are important in nutrition. The future will add to the list. Still other minerals can affect us. Arsenic in large enough amounts kills. Moderate amounts can cause cancer. Traces appear harmless.

I have mentioned the villains cadmium and lead. There is also mercury poisoning. Radium is hazardous to health and life in strong concentrations. Many more minerals pass through us regularly, disposed of by our bodies with no harm that we know of. That appraisal, too, is only as good as today's knowledge. The potential for good or for evil of many more minerals will be better known as time goes on. Meantime, get those we know you need.

Now let's turn to other nutrients that belong in this summary.

CARBOHYDRATES (CHO)

Carbohydrates have us in a perpetual dither and cost us millions of dollars a year. In spite of everything written about white sugar and refined white flour making us fat and undermining health by displacing good nutrients in our daily habits, the two continue as our main sources of CHO.

Carbohydrates comprise 25 to 50 percent of most people's total food and beverage intake. Add to this nearly equal amounts of questionable fats and this combination leaves many of us in affluent malnutrition.

We not only waste billions better spent on more healthful food, but more billions trying to undo the results of eating the wrong foods. *We* raise the meat prices with our run on fat-marbled steaks and chops. *We* invest in diet books and diet fads. *We* pay for carbohydrate charts, low-carbohydrate sauces, ready-made foods marketed to catch us when we decide to avoid CHO.

In sum, carbohydrate intake has the whole nation off nutritional balance, along with calorie intake (1 gram CHO equals 4 calories). But common sense must rule. Carbohydrates derived from grains and root vegetables provide most of the world's people their chief energy sources. We can't do without CHO any more than we can, for long, abuse our bodies with overdoses of it.

You don't have to swing back and forth between CHO deprivation when conscience gets the upper hand and carbohydrate binges when you don't give a damn. Veer away from worthless foods that now fill your body. Make room for a regimen that isn't so Spartan that it sets you up for failure. To free yourself of the overload–starve syndrome, keep reading.

FAT

Fat contains about 9 calories per gram. Give or take a frankfurter or well-marbled steak, the average fat content in our highly touted American diet actually is 50 percent. That's far too high.

Apart from danger to our hearts and arteries, cholesterol buildup and other fat-linked problems, the same situation exists with too much fat as with too much CHO. A diet heavy in fat, like one heavy in carbohydrates, simply doesn't leave room for what you need to achieve a healthy, vigorous body.

Our sweet teeth, fast-food tastes, faddism and bouts with conscience lead us a merry existence, true, but we must have some fat. The Eskimos proved it. On heavy exercise and unprocessed, unchemicalized foods in a rugged, *healthy* environment, large quantities of fats and oils are *not* unhealthy. Studies of modern Italian diets (20 to 30 percent fat as opposed to our 40 to 50 percent) prove the same thing.

As we nudge you away from convenience foods, bakery foods, fatty foods, white flour and white sugar, we must remind you that excess polyunsaturates are also not the answer. Our diets should not be over 20 percent in polyunsaturates.

My appraisal is that you should get 10 to 15 percent of your daily diet in polyunsaturates and about 10 percent in saturates, while at the same time being certain you get the other needed nutrients. Use cold-pressed fresh oils. Use fresh vegetables as much as possible. Rely on whole grains, seeds and nuts, as well as lots of fish and some fresh meat. In selecting meats, stick to those relatively low in saturated fat content.

PROTEINS

Americans who say rich, juicy steaks are the nation's number one sex food are wrong. Sorry. Engorgement of the pelvic area by steak, spices, alcohol and other urinary-tract irritants may make you aware of your genital zone, and if available sex takes your mind off the problem, there's no quarreling with it. But if you think the food that caused the itch improves your prowess, forget it. Those who rarely tank up on such foods, including groups that eat little or no meat at all, do just as well and better. Vegetarians make good lovers without a taste of meat. If you crave endurance for many years of pleasurable sex play, that takes us right back to the Caucasus.

We know the protein foods. Fish, cheese, milk, yogurt, roe, eggs (don't overdo) and many other foods provide protein. Plan 25 percent of your calories around eating foods from *good* protein sources. For reference, 1 gram of protein equals 4 calories.

Add to your protein sources by mixing foods, as we've suggested. Armenians are artists at stretching meat. They can serve a dozen people by chopping a pound of lamb into a variable mix of fruits, vegetables or both; adding nuts, seeds or both; creating memorable novelties, practicing economy and offering high nutrition at low relative cost.

Any meat will do. Your cleverness can provide a feast for a dozen or more, all palatable, nutritious and novel enough to draw cheers. What you can do with meats you can also do with cheese and/or grains.

Use meat to stuff fruit and fruit to stuff meat. Add nuts. And if you find the idea of grains supplying proteins revolutionary, you should know that grains provide half the world's protein supply. They're not novel at all as protein food.

I have kept my remarks on carbohydrates, fats and proteins brief because we have much more ground to cover.

I would like to end this important section of the book with summary observations. Following them, we have included a chart that summarizes the average vitamin and mineral recommendations I'd like to make.

My Caucasus research convinces me that substances there that contribute to longevity are chromium; the antioxidants C and E; zinc and fiber foods (see Chapter 9); B complex, especially in their yogurt and acidophilus milk; vitamin A, especially in their fish oils, liver and organ meats; and their abundance of vitamin-A rich vegetables, apricots, plums, walnuts, almonds, sunflower and sesame seeds, grape concentrate (*petmez*), garlics, fish roe, seafood, whole grain-cereals (especially bulgur, oats, millet, barley and whole-grain rice), plus a wide range of herbs and botanicals.

For bone youthfulness (saving sex for Chapter 7), we might include vanadium foods, chromium and zinc foods, vitamin-D foods, absorbable calcium, botanicals and good sources of vitamins A, E, C and iron which work together for absorption of calcium.

For heart and blood-vessel youthfulness, we've suggested vitamin-C foods, fiber foods, unrefined grains, roe, fish, seeds, nuts, fresh vegetables and lecithin, vitamin E, iodine and chromium foods. Avoid getting too much fat from eggs. Mix liberally among all these sources without overdoing on any. In the same way, we have small amounts of vitamin K-supplying foods, foods supplying us with the B complex, B_6 and magnesium to make it work and zinc foods. And here we say again that *moderate* quantities of meat are not only adequate for protein balance but advisable for healthy hearts and arteries.

External youthful appearance is assisted by thyroid- and pituitary-gland helpers, protein and vitamin-rich foods emphasizing especially vitamins A, B_6, C and F for the pituitary, modest iodine sources, iron, chromium, magnesium and zinc. As mentioned earlier, regular and adequate supplies of vitamin A are also necessary for sound teeth, bones, skin, eyes and hair, each important to youthful appearance. Don't forget, too, the recipe for correction or prevention of gray hair: inositol, PABA and pantothenate.

Brain-benefitting youthfulness comes from time-release vitamin-C capsules plus botanicals and foods rich in vitamin C; from niacin (here, too, we suggest the value of time-release capsules); and from prescriptions for niacin, B_{12}, C, thiamine, folic acid, B_6, magnesium, glutamic acid or hydrochloric acid drops (especially for the elderly), riboflavin, pantothenic acid, and, where poor diet has led to depression, biotin, tryptophane (an essential amino acid), all known amino acids and adequate protein. You also need adequate potassium, lecithin (phospholipids, choline and inositol as building blocks) and enough unsaturated oil, as we've said, to make the lecithin work.

Remembering that circumstances alter individual cases, here are:

Seven Sensible Steps for Longer Lifetime Nutrition

1. Take between-meal pick-me-ups such as acidophilus tablets, also *kefir* grains, particularly good for dieters who can't fit

yogurt into their schedules but who should avoid excess calories and carbohydrates.

2. Add daily time-release niacin (nicotinic acid) to improve brain performance of the elderly and peripheral or leg/arm circulation performance.

3. Take time-release vitamin-C capsules, which are a definite aid to health, especially for people who must avoid citrus.

4. Find and use a reliable vanadium source for better bones, remembering that most American gelatin and bone-meal sources are deficient in vanadium.

5. See that your diet includes a chromium source to restore reserves most Americans have lost by age thirty. Neglected in most dietary regimens, chromium helps us retain youthfulness.

6. Use garlic, preferably the fresh clove, another rich nutrient too often neglected in American diets.

7. Increase your knowledge and use of herbs and botanicals. Formulas vary as people and needs do. I have mentioned zinc sources and mineral-rich teas (cloves to buy *fresh,* to break or grind) for chromium to drink alone or add to mint, rose hips, alfalfa or comfrey. Use new herbs and botanicals sparingly, either in teas or soups. Take herbs and botanicals seriously. We will have more to say about their qualities and uses in Chapter 6.

Before we look at the chart summarizing my modest supplementation recommendations for average adults, I should acknowledge my personal frustration, no doubt matched by yours, that no manufacturer ever seems to produce in a single pill all of what we need for supplementation. This occurs partly because needs vary so much. But I am convinced that supplementation is *necessary* every day to compensate for depleted soils, delays in marketing, processing, and so on, which rob us daily. I hope that manufacturers will explore this fact and make a serious effort to produce the chart formula in a single capsule or pill—at most, in two—remembering how much better so many of these vitamins and minerals work for us when taken together. So saying, I want to add that I hope research will continue so that the holes in the chart—where no recommendations are made because we don't know enough—will soon be filled.

Daily Supplements Recommended by McQ-WMS

Caution: Consult your doctor before using. These are average adult recommendations and he may suggest variations for specific conditions. DO NOT USE FOR CHILDREN OR INFANTS.

VITAMIN A *4,000 units*
VITAMIN B_1 (thiamine) *2 mg.*
VITAMIN B_2 (riboflavin) *2.5 mg.*
VITAMIN B_3 (niacin) *15 mg.*
VITAMIN B_6 (pyridoxine) *3 mg. (up to 100 mg. in cases of deficiency)*
PANTOTHENATE *36 mg.*
PABA *100 mg.*
INOSITOL *1,500-3,000 mg. (19-grain lecithin/1,200 mg.)*
CHOLINE *1,500-2,000 mg.*
BIOTIN *1 mg.*
FOLIC ACID *.1 mg.*
VITAMIN B_{12} (cobalomine) *5 mcg.*
VITAMIN C *500 mg. (time-release)*
VITAMIN D_3 *400 units*
VITAMIN E *100 mg.*
VITAMIN F
VITAMIN K *2 mg.*
VITAMIN P
VITAMIN Q
VITAMIN U

BROMINE
CALCIUM *1 g. (elderly: 1-2 g.)*
CHLORINE *.5 g.*
CHROMIUM *2 mg.*
COPPER *2 mg.*
FLUORINE *.5 mg.*
IODINE *.1-.2 mg.*
IRON *10-12 mg.*
MAGNESIUM *50-100 mg.*
PHOSPHORUS *1 g.*
POTASSIUM
SODIUM
VANADIUM
ZINC *10-15 mg.*

units = international units or I.U.
mg. = milligrams
mcg. = micrograms
g. = grams

6. Herbs, Botanicals and You

There are more than enough definitions for botanicals and herbs. Ignoring them all, I think of the two more or less interchangeably. If that be heresy, let the naturalists make the most of it.

We are concerned in this chapter with natural growing things with medicinal value, nutritional value or both. Our concern doesn't suggest that you graze in the meadow to get these values, although that makes more sense than grazing in supermarkets for worthless refined sugar and flour and products containing them.

Leaving others to define herbs and botanicals, I'd like to define antioxidants or at least help you understand something about them. The two best-known antioxidants are vitamin C and the vitamin E group. Outside the body, whatever retards oxidation (rusting, for example) can be called an antioxidant. In the body, oxidation is part of the continual process by which oxygen, carried through the bloodstream, unites with other substances as oxidases (oxidizing enzymes), as part of the continual cycle of cellular development and cellular breakdown that keeps our bodies healthy.

Vitamin E's effectiveness as a body-balancing antioxidant was proved in Dr. Evans' pioneering work at Berkeley. Vitamin C's antioxidant activity has satisfied many of us of the high value of this much-attacked fighter for health and longevity.

More recently, there has been some provocative work at Stanford University on cell survival in laboratory cultures. The Stanford results, verified through independent duplications of the same basic work, indicate that people have natural built-in time clocks; that human cells are programmed for fifty plus or minus ten dividings, the exact number probably depending on variable genetic and environmental factors. (Obviously, if something kills us first we don't get the full allotment.) But given normal conditions (whatever they are), the Stanford work seems to say we are programmed for threescore and ten, give or take a few years.

I don't deride the Stanford work. It is a milestone in cellular research. But it leaves us with mysteries if we are to accept from it that, no matter what frantic efforts we make to live longer, once the fifty plus or minus ten dividings have taken place, it's all over for us.

My practice and experience make me reject that premise entirely. For starters, back at Berkeley a successor named Leslie Packer recently performed his own version of the Stanford experiments, significantly adding only vitamin E (antioxidant) to his culture. Just as significantly, he produced not fifty plus or minus ten cell dividings but more than a hundred, approximating the centenarian state in human life.

This extension of Dr. Evans's vitamin E discovery is at least as exciting as our original work at Berkeley. It is something very tangible to hold onto as we try to understand things happening in the Caucasus that are not happening here.

My effort to convey the important findings noted just above has necessarily skimmed lightly over a very heavy subject. What you might visualize now is a pipe so rusted within by oxidation, and so narrowed by the buildups of minerals and chemicals passing through it, that it finally fills solidly with matter, becomes blocked and totally impassable. Now visualize an artery that has become so clogged by cholesterol and other sterols and chemical/mineral deposits as to become blocked and impassable. That comparison should enable you to see the value of antioxidants which prevent buildups and keep the passageways clear. Apply this reasoning to the miles of human arteries, veins and capillaries, the vital network in our life-maintenance process, and we have made our point. I firmly believe in antioxidants as little understood blood-vessel detergents that prolong life.

Antioxidants have been a prime constituent of the herbal/botanical recipes my husband and I have used with great success in patient care. By careful analysis of symptoms and equally careful applications of combinations of natural juices from greens, roots, barks and florals—some our own inventions and others older than written history—we have helped a great number of sick people who had been given up or left unaided by others.

Can our results be taken seriously? After all, science insists on definite validation procedures before it accepts a claimed development as proved. To establish validity, we must have a test group and a control group. I give you the mixed populations of the

Caucasus as one of those groups and our Westernized peoples as the other. The Caucasus group, as I mentioned, produce 65 per 100,000 population at or above centenarian age. Some of them reach what we consider extraordinary ages. We produce in the United States some 3 per 100,000 with no such extreme ages.

We're not describing an experiment now, nor anything new. The Caucasus peoples have been doing their old-age thing for centuries. We, of course, have been at our processed, chemicalized fodder long enough to hurl a mass behavioristic roadblock in the way of our otherwise great progress in science and medicine.

We know all about our way of life. This book is trying to tell you about theirs: natural, unprocessed foods; a diet low in fatty red meats; emphasis on fresh fruits, fresh vegetables and whole-grain cereals and breads, fiber foods of special side benefit (see Chapter 9)—all this within a regimen of dedicated daily exercise (Chapter 8). Anything else? Yes, the Caucasians have a fondness for adding herbs and botanicals to literally everything they prepare. This habit provides the Caucasus people with a continuing supply of antioxidants in their varied salads and through their lifelong preference for mixing foods. Remember those half-dozen salads Kegan and I were served with *each* Caucasus meal?

Their habit of spiking everything with herbs is a product of respect for the medicinal benefits in herbs, observed and enjoyed there for centuries. Kegan brought these observations into his laboratory. Once he had broken down the values that made those herbs work, he turned Armenian folklore into successful treatments of conditions labelled hopeless before we saw them.

How do I dare call herbs and botanicals a key link in the Caucasus chain of longevity? Something in them plainly does the job. I have concluded that that something is many more natural antioxidants, perhaps in the form of enzyme antioxidases, than science and medicine have been capable of breaking down and identifying up to now. What is clear to me is that peoples who make fresh herbs and botanicals a habit benefit in years and health and incidentally, in sexual vigor, from the cumulative antioxidant activities occurring in their bodies due to natural sources.

Stuff and nonsense? No, the stuff in today's medical practice is some of the flood tide of synthetic-chemical nostrums rolling into us as alleged cures and palliatives. The stuff in pills for diabetes, for instance, for some time administered to save lives, is suddenly thought to contribute to heart-related death within five years in many patients.

Also, statistics now available comparing cholera patients

who are given the full course of treatment both with and without administration of chloramphenicol show that patients off the drug do just as well as those on the drug.

Further, evidence in doctors' hands for some years has curtailed sharply our once free-and-easy prescriptions of the wonder drugs. Too often they lead to such side effects as potentially fatal allergy. Too, we have steadily discovered that germ strains are prone to retreat under attack by wonder drugs, only to return immune to them.

We wonder about wonder drugs as we cut down and phase out their use in diabetes, in digestive illnesses, in "preventive" medicine, in treating the obese, in allergy and elsewhere. The great hopes for the wonder drugs have faded.

As they decline in use, what's to replace them? Some say more wonder drugs. But the explosion of products from the chemical factories is already causing synergistic problems. Patients are being found to persist in using what one doctor prescribed as they add what Doctor No. 2 prescribes and even what Doctors No. 3 and No. 4 prescribe. As a consequence, we are finding that Doctor No. 4 didn't know about what the others prescribed (or, too often, didn't know that the *combination* of prescriptions was a loaded gun).

New pills are not the answer in my judgment. Proved natural remedies have endured the test of time throughout the world. More such items are being consumed today than are chemicals from factories. Even today in the United States about half the constituents of products we purchase as medicines are either herbs or botanicals or products inspired by them.

When people realize they have been (not deliberately) misled as science has misled itself through reliance on pill chemistry to sustain or restore the body to health, more of us will sensibly turn back to active herbs, botanicals and vegetables for natural preventive medicine.

In this turnabout we're behind others. Chairman Mao Tsetung started a revival in China in 1959. He signalled a return to herbal medicines at a time when Western influences had nearly wiped out China's ancient herbal arts. Doctors recently sent there by the American Medical Association reported in JAMA that botanical treatment seems to be working fine.

I have studied documented cases of infants from Vietnam with reported diseases, some fatal, beyond medical knowledge. No pills from our present best chemistry seemed helpful. Doctors finally turned to healthy donors for an old natural remedy, mother's milk. It brought miraculous recoveries.

This lies close to something else observed in recent medical reports. For years, women have been told not to gain over fifteen pounds in pregnancy. We all grew up on that. *At a recent conference, doctors revised the figure to 24 pounds.* Medicine is not infallible. We plod along learning, making mistakes, doing our best with what we know until we know better.

The blush is off the roseate notion that mankind can find nirvana in pills. We have come full circle with the conclusion that pills (including The Pill) replace natural methods at human peril. We've made this full circle, ironically, after letting our growing and grazing lands deplete. To turn to nature for help today, we are constrained to grow our fresh supplies in window boxes, in postage-stamp garden patches, fields next to factories and wherever else we might till ourselves, to gain some salvation before it's too late.

I am far from alone in using herbs in my practice. Recently, British herbal physicians won the right to have their pharmacopeia given equal weight with allopathic and homeopathic pharmacopeias. Americans well eventually follow. We have nowhere else to go when we inevitably surrender the unreality of living off pills.

I've already covered the manner in which chemicals in our foods add up to dangers for us. When one adds pharmaceutical chemistry to food chemistry, is it logical that the total effect will be greater danger of synergistic symptoms rather than less? The answer is obvious. In my judgment, the total of medical chemistry and food chemistry in our bodies will eventually be recognized as one of mankind's saddest mistakes.

When you consider this major difference between our way of life and the chemical-free Caucasus way, the decision to adapt their dietary and exercise habits into our own regimens is irresistible.

If all this has interested you in botanicals, there are books good and not so good that help us recognize their qualities and grow them. Intelligent readers can separate the sensational from the convincing. Dabble in fresh herbs for food preparation and your results will draw you to experiment further, even if slowly at first. So doing, you'll find new taste pleasures and new nutritional values. And you'll have taken another of the group of steps this book suggests for better health and longevity.

Can habits change? Here's a very simple illustration. After four years away in World War II, a patient of mine saw his father drinking unsweetened black coffee. Before he had left, his father took cream and four heaping teaspoons of sugar in his coffee. The son asked, "How did this happen?" His father explained, "They told me to get my weight down. I couldn't do it. Then one night I heard Walter Winchell talking about his weight. Someone advised him to eliminate a quarter of a teaspoon of sugar from his coffee until he was used to the taste, then cut out another quarter teaspoon, until he finally got it down to nothing. I did that and did the same thing with the cream. It worked." His father's final comment was, "And you know, son, *that's* [the black coffee] a very nice drink."

You can reduce use of refined white sugar the same way, a bit at a time until you confound the sugar interests by breaking your addiction. Also, you can break with refined white flour, if you do your own baking, mixing decreasing amounts of refined flour with increasing amounts of whole-wheat flour until you've switched over altogether. A woman patient of mine has done just that. Today she bakes magnificent chocolate cakes with whole-wheat flour and plans to begin substituting carob for the chocolate as a further health benefit. Her gingerbreads, made with whole-wheat flour and dark molasses, are a delight.

Accept this: It took miracle after miracle for mankind to begin to live on this planet. For mankind to survive and develop in his tropical Eden, nature provided vegetation with the power to help do the job. The power is still there. Nature's storehouse of botanicals is still available as nutrition and medicine.

There has been no conspiracy to deprive us of this birthright in order to sell pills and patent medicines. We simply "advanced" ourselves into our unhappy state. Medicine's stunning achievements have been larded with unproductive and even dangerous products. As consumers, we were eager to believe what science was eager to believe it had produced for our salvation. Now we must give nature another try. She has been neglected too long, except by too few of us who have made nutrition our life's work.

I would like to finish this chapter with some remarks about some, but hardly all of the botanicals you should know. This will not be a complete work on herbs. I have picked a few of my favorites to introduce you to the subject, to open the door a bit. I'll mention the medicinal values of some and the value of adding others generously to salads, soups and general cookery.

You'll love some immediately. You'll learn to use others. Still others you may reject for personal taste reasons. The important thing is to incorporate herbs and botanicals into what I've been calling a total package of steps for better health and longer life. Consider this group:

ASARUM

This plant, with its heart-shaped or pointed green leaves, does poorly in gardens, thrives in moist woodland areas. I prefer Japanese or European varieties for my patients. Minimum amounts are effective. Small amounts are always a good idea in introducing any herb. With asarum, an herbal doctor should supervise. Do not dabble with it on your own.

In my practice, asarum powder has reduced uric-acid levels, as in gout. I have helped arthritis sufferers, even in cases of rheumatoid arthritis, reducing the rheumatoid factor all the way down to zero in some cases with asarum-powder capsules. This remedy seems most effective in the age range of thirty to sixty in arthritis, rheumatism, hypertrophic arthritis, rheumatism and gallbladder trouble associated with liver abnormalities. I have seen it give good results in bursitis, sciatica, stiff necks, some headache conditions and such neuromuscular-skeletal complaints as neck-shoulder-hand syndrome.

I used asarum to return bricklayers to their jobs. They had been in so much pain that they couldn't work. I used it to cure a noted violinist of neck-shoulder-hand syndrome which threatened to halt a great career, and again to send a seamstress (she sewed beads on thousand-dollar dresses) back to her stitching. In these and other cases, asarum worked where earlier remedies had failed, giving the outcome the appearance of a miracle to those unfortunate patients whose careers and livelihoods were threatened.

Persons used to aspirin seem to do well with asarum, but those with chronic weak stomachs or nervous digestive complaints are best advised to take asarum under special care of an herbal physician. Remember, no self-treatment.

An observation relative to asarum is that, long before chemists hit on cortisone, Mexicans in two areas where yams grow were consuming the large roots after boiling them and perhaps with other special handling, apparently aware that the juice ingested from the roots sometimes had anti-arthritic properties. Asarum, which has similar properties, has been a favorite in our laboratory. Components of asarum are known to chemists. In contrast to aspirin, which sometimes provokes side effects and whose aid is temporary, asarum, correctly administered, seems to *build* results, providing longer-lasting help.

BASIL

This herb can cost you from two cents a month to two cents a day, depending on how much you use. A reason such herbs are given so little official sanction as medicines is that they can scarcely be classified as profit makers.

Basil (*Ocimum basilicum*) grows tender green leaves. In the

Caucasus, Persia, India, Chile, Java and the United States, its fresh leaves are mixed with other greens, go into salads, soups, stews and sauces and make beverages like tea. Dried leaves can be bought in most stores.

Basil is as aromatic as mint. It is as medicinally effective as clove and eucalyptus, and is useful against nervous collapse and asthenia (lack of strength), nervous insomnia, vertigo, stomach spasms, intestinal grippe, pulmonary problems, general pain, distress and anxiety. (This is not the full list.)

I have used basil with magical success for sick, choking children after their pediatricians had tried routine treatment, including antibiotics, without success. In just a few hours basil teas in hot extracts reduced adenoidal signs and symptoms, fever and malaise. When basil is used, even recurrent cases have been observed to get well and stay well. Sinuses, ears and breathing can become normal and trouble-free by use of this remedy provided by nature. The mothers of my young patients have told me that when they see first signs of new colds these days they quickly give basil tea. The signs disappear.

BRANS

We're hearing more of the role of these foods as fiber, or roughage. That's fine. Brans can be purchased widely in all wheat-bran forms without added chemicals, salt or sugar. Rice bran and rice-bran products can be bought with no additives, as can unmanipulated barley, millet, corn and oats—all whole grains and whole-grain flours.

The whole-grain, bran-rich flours, bought in health-food stores if not available in regular markets, should be used instead of refined white flours. If no store nearby has them, you can order them by mail from Eastern sources, more in the Middle West, Texas and California. If you hadn't thought of brans as herbs, think again.

Locate sources of natural mill products. Get catalogues. Discuss these products with other health-minded people and swap sources with them. (In recommending such sources, let me assure you that I have no connection with any of them, except as a customer.) If no one can tell you where these sources are located, read the ads in nutrition magazines. You can also trace them from their labels on products in health-food stores. Buying direct is enough of a cost-saving incentive to make the effort worthwhile.

At my suggestion, some of my patients have purchased their own home-sized mills, buying only whole grains and reducing them as needed. Not a bad idea at all.

Here's how the most familiar grains stack up in fiber value: wheat-bran flakes provide 10.3 g. fiber per 100 g./edible portion; rice bran, 12 g.; alfalfa seed, 7.5 g.; carob powder, 5.05 g.; chick-peas, 5.3 g.; lentils, 3.7 g.; whole flaxseed, 4.9 g.; millet, 3.5 g. Try mixing the ones you don't enjoy by themselves. For example, add split peas (1.2 g.) to improve the taste of others.

There's another good reason to mix grains. Most grains are individually deficient in certain protein values. Mixing adds the values in one to those in the other(s). Remember the nutritional provender of brans. In addition to fiber values, as charts indicate, brans have potassium, manganese, zinc, iron, niacin and more.

Caution: Some people, such as those with already developed ulcers, hemorrhoids and diverticulitis, must avoid brans and all hard fibers, confining their intake to soft fibers such as pectin. A doctor's guidance is necessary for these cases.

CHAMOMILE (German: *Matricaria chamomilla;* Italian: *Anthemis nobilis)*

These species are alike in some ways and dissimilar in others. Let's take them one at a time, German first because I know that many aware Americans send to Germany for theirs.

I have seen it help against indigestion or malassimilation, particularly where these are associated with diagnosed gallbladder conditions. Taken as tea (tisane), infused up to an hour, sipped hot and quite bitter, it quiets digestive disturbances and calms the sipper as it perks him up. I take it myself. The results are excellent.

It's also helpful as an antispasmodic, gentle nerve tonic, especially for discomforted infants. As shown by European tests with controls, it has wound-healing, anti-inflammatory properties. Used externally, it is effective on old wounds, bad eczemas, urticaria and pruritis of the vulva or genitalia, as well as ulcers of the legs.

Italian chamomile is better-known in the Mediterranean, Caucasus and Middle East. It has many of the virtues I've just described. It appears to be anti-anemic and seems to help against grippe. It aids discomforted infants and is useful in skin and digestive conditions just as the German variety. One also sees it deployed effectively against nervous conditions, menopausal troubles, headaches, migraines, neuralgias and vertigo. American doctors should know that it can challenge any commercial pills in this regard. Externally, it is used as the German variety is, with good results.

Both are taken alike: 5 to 10 "heads" (each smaller than a bachelor's button) are infused to make a cup of tea. Italian chamomile is also powdered and sometimes appears as an essence.

Externally, it is used as a decoction, applied or rubbed on as doctors direct, or used gently as an oil base, soak or mini-bath for an affected part. I have heard of chamomile's effectiveness, too, as an antirheumatic soak or bath. (Sex-minded readers may be interested to learn that such soaks have been advanced for aphrodisiac purposes with allegedly interesting results. I have not used chamomile this way and cannot comment.)

FENUGREEK (*Chaman*) (No connection with cumin or curry)

Popular in the Caucasus, it is also grown in Persia, Egypt, nearby Africa and India (where many Caucasus recipes have found their way). Like many other Caucasus items, fenugreek is suspected of having originated in the Orient in antiquity.

Fenugreek has a remarkable aroma, disliked in many places not used to it. It is the distinguishing item of *basterma*, a delicious, unforgettable Armenian dried meat sausage. For centuries, Kegan's sources indicated that it was a restorative for malnourished people.

What's in it? Much more than lore. Modern chemistry and animal research reveal fenugreek as a remarkable source for lecithin, choline and phytins, plus a derivative of niacin or vitamin P. Thus, what we know today about fenugreek demonstrates the wisdom of the ages. It has been shown to have high value among plant items with nutritional content.

It has been used to improve neuromuscular powers (strength, endurance, energy), and has enjoyed a reputation as a sex-power aid. Today, we know it contains an unusual steroid-saponin compound nearly identical to a sex-related chemical hydrolyzed from the Mexican yam, diosgenin, the source of cortisone and the sex hormones, testosterone and progesterone. This information is from Prof. R. Paris, department head at the University of France and a leading *materia medica* expert and botanist. If you infer from this that you should cultivate a taste for fenugreek (or cultivate it if you can), you're right.

GARLIC (French: *ail*)

I'll take time for just one historic fact from the rich background of this botanical. When cholera, typhus, influenza and black plague become epidemic in many parts of this world, the price of garlic escalates tenfold and disappears from the market overnight. History shows that the prominent survivors of these onslaughts have been those who managed to get their hands on enough garlic to take some daily with liquor. This was in contrast to the thousands who died in epidemics.

I call garlic a natural antibiotic. That's not a fancy of mine. Garlic is in the *Liliaceae* (lily) family. Some of its relatives offer sulfur derivatives such as Americans find present in sulfonamides and penicillins.

Garlic has been a Caucasus favorite since antiquity. From early childhood, more is consumed in that part of the world than anywhere else of record. There are garlic sauces, garlic-laced gravies, stews, soups and salads. Meats and cheeses are garlic-juiced or cloved; fish, bread, pilaf—in fact, everything but coffee and desserts gets garlic.

In addition to regular intake, Caucasus peoples take enormous amounts at the first sign of any illness. Unlike Americans who grudgingly take garlic capsules after developing heart disease, diabetes, hypercholesterolemia, high blood pressure, piles or varicose veins, as a group of some forty nationalities, Caucasus peoples take garlic and generally avoid these diseases.

French scientists, for the most part, have detected in garlic antiseptics, vermifuges, diuretics and compounds effective against chest diseases such as pneumonia and bronchitis. Much is known about garlic and why, taken early and in quantity, it may indeed benefit many people in many circumstances.

I can tell you from my own experience that one clove (not a bunch) taken at night makes hemorrhoids and recurrent constipation vanish. I have had a good percentage of success with it. Personally, I dislike taking much more than that or even taking it daily unless you are beset by cholera-diarrhea or an epidemic of plague. Caucasus daily use is, however, quite healthful—in normal habit a touch in soups, lamb and staples, a rub in salads. Those touches and rubs add up.

Before scoffing, here's a suggestion: Instead of drenching your foods in butter, ketchup, or your favorite kitchen sauces, mustard mixes, and so on, you might benefit your health as well as your palate by subtle garlic use. As a condiment, garlic offers benefits not unlike those of its cousins, chives, shallots, scallions and onions.

GINGER (*Zingiber officinale*)

In the Orient, the Caucasus, along the trade routes to western Europe, in the Philippines and exotic Tahiti, ginger is noted for prevention of impotence, as an antiseptic and a tonic.

In beverages, nonalcoholic and as ginger beer or brandy, it probably reaches the urinary system, benefitting the kidney, bladder and the male prostate, and very possibly having a good effect against early impotency.

It has definite hind-end values for man and beast. As a topical rectal treatment, it aids the pelvic area. In racehorses, it is a known remedy for drooping tail and helps provide a "healthy horse" appearance.

Externally, it is widely used in liniment formulas—with cyprus, for instance, and with rosemary and origan of the mint family, which seem to have little potency by themselves. Ginger is used with a few drops of turpentine as a tincture for rubbing on rheumatic and arthritic areas. Internally, varied tinctures or extracts containing ginger can relieve aches and pains of rheumatic diseases or angina accompanied by edema (swelling).

Ginger has antiseptic, tonic, stimulant properties. It has a record of relief of malassimilation, indigestion, gaseous dyspepsia and diarrhea-type fevers. It also enjoys a reputation for prevention of contagious diseases.

Its known components include an oleoresin called zingiberol, various phenolic compounds, zingiberene and zingerone. All are from fresh roots. People everywhere enjoy it as a beverage, condiment, pick-me-up. It braces sauces and foods. Some people like it in a hot drink, some cold.

Unlike aspirin, it attacks pain and discomfort without stomach upset, bleeding, dopeyness and sleeplessness. Ginger possesses no detectable salicylic compounds. It is neither willow nor wintergreen, from which salicylate use began.

I do not advise living on ginger or on any of the mentioned botanicals. Let nobody develop an all-garlic, all-ginger or garlic-ginger diet. It will be as unbalanced as those already attacked. But moderate experimentation and use of all these and other treasures from nature's own storehouse, the earth, will lead to many benefits. But if you are somehow troubled by taking any of these botanicals (through allergy or some individuality of makeup), discontinue use and see your doctor.

GINSENG (*Panax schinseng*)

Gin signifies man-root in English because some specimens resemble the human figure. Likewise, from the Greek word *pan*, *panax* stands for remedy (panacea). Ginseng has a history as broad and long as world trade routes. A single example: Korean ox-drivers and cow-herders dose up on it when they can find it, becoming romantic and gay. Ginseng grows in Korea, Siberia and parts of the Caucasus. An American variety, once exported to the Orient, fell from favor here. It seems that distance lends enchantment to the effectiveness of aphrodisiacs.

Ginseng contains a little essential oil, best encapsulated or rendered in liquid extract because the roots dry quickly. It takes a lot of roots to make a capsule since each root contains only a trace amount. Ginseng also boasts resin, starch, sterols; triterpenic sapogenins, glucides, which some define as arabinose; glucose and rhamnose. It also contains some thiamine and riboflavin.

Experiments I have read about seem to show that feeding considerable ginseng to a female castrated rat may induce signs of estrus (heat). An experiment in 1960–61 by a Professor Petune concluded that ginseng can have "stimulant effect" on the nervous system, defraying fatigue.

I have also read that a certain undefined hormone said to be in some batches may act on its users somewhat as a hormone shot does. Some of my patients have taken it on their own. I haven't found any response in them from it, neither feminization nor any other kind of response. But patients of both sexes have said it makes them feel healthy, joyous and benign toward others.

In spite of its popularity as a rejuvenator since at least the first century, I can't say I have seen it perform even mundane miracles, let alone rejuvenation. It is not much used in the Caucasus in my observation. I continue to believe that the good health Caucasians enjoy is from adherence to the regimen of living habits we are describing, not to ginseng. Sorry about that.

HOT PEPPERS

Most green peppers turn red and hotter to the tongue if allowed to mature. U.S. peppers are annuals, growing almost anywhere in good soil. People who shun peppers should know that the red variety provides 464 percent of the MDR of vitamin C; 430 percent vitamin A; 23 percent niacin; 22 percent riboflavin; 17 percent thiamine; 6 percent phosphorus and some potassium. A raw hot chili pepper contains 103 mg. vitamin C. A medium pimento from the can has 36 mg. vitamin C.

In Western medicine, pepper (*Piper nigrum*) has been used with cinnamon to cure migraine headaches, as an antiblennorrhagic (discharge of pus) and as a curative in certain stomach and intestinal disorders.

There's a story about an American-born doctor setting up a practice in the Caucasus. He observed workers in the fields devouring hot peppers at lunch, wolfing them down with other equally spicy, hot foods. Then he saw them go home and have more of the same at supper. When they failed to come to him with their insides in an uproar, he gave up and moved away. Where diet is highly spiced with hot peppers, as in the Caucasus, Egypt, Thailand, Austria, Hungary, Bulgaria and elsewhere, people don't suffer from stomach ulcers, leg ulcers, blood clots and other circulatory disorders. And constipation and hemorrhoids are nearly unknown.

Bangkok physicians recently speculated that peppery diet is behind their people's freedom from blood clots and circulatory ailments. Two groups were experimentally fed Oriental noodles, one group with and the other without hot peppers and peppery sauces. Laboratory testing showed better performance in withstanding blood clotting in the peppery dieters than the others for the first thirty minutes after eating, after which both were the same or normal. It all seems to indicate that Americans suffering from coronary obstruction, varicose veins, leg clotting and hemorrhoids, as well as conditions associated with clotting, stroke or apoplexy, might benefit from a change of diet such as we are suggesting.

We say again that more botanicals and a less refined diet may be the difference between the ages and health stages we attain and those in the Caucasus.

LEGUMES (Edible: beans, chick-peas, lentils, peas)

Legumes came out of the Orient, were smuggled along the caravan routes and settled down to become a mainstay in the Caucasus diet before moving across the Black Sea and west to Bulgaria, thence our way. Some will tell you bean eating is the secret of strength, sexuality and longevity, with or without yogurt, cheeses, meats or fish in good times.

I'll just touch on the high vitamin content in legumes: the B-complex vitamins, especially pantothenate, niacin, thiamine and some carotene (vitamin-A precursor); tocopherols (vitamin E and the antioxidant group); vitamin-D traces; and some steroid saponin. Yes, and high-protein content: glucides, lecithin and lipids (oils).

There are many types with many shadings of taste: green beans (*haricot* to the French), soybeans, peas, fava, the lentils, many varieties of faseoli. Most provide youth-giving lecithin. Legumes are good nutrition for man or beast.

LUZERNE (Lucerne; Lucern; Alfalfa)

This forage crop grows throughout the temperate zones. Alfalfa and other sprouts are becoming increasingly popular as people recognize in them opportunities to have something super-fresh in their salads and soups. Sprouting your own is an excellent idea for the reasons I shall give.

Luzerne, as the French call it, contains vitamins K_1, C, D, E and carotene. Sprouts were used for centuries before K_1, the coagulation vitamin, was discovered in 1939. Alfalfa is mineral-rich, with varying amounts of iron, potassium and phosphate, depending on where the roots grow. These are deep growing roots, capable of sucking up more or less whatever minerals they please.

One use of luzerne is as a tisane against early arthritis. It can also be useful against development of anemia. Its mineral-gobbling roots make it valuable for bone healing. It is also known as a recalcifiant and reconstituent.

In the Caucasus we found big sprout users, and this mineral store, taken for a lifetime, is believed partly responsible for the excellent teeth even the oldsters have in their mouths.

MULBERRY

In the Greater Caucasus mulberries are eaten in great quantities. Silkworms get the leaf as part of the area's silk business, but the people get the berries. The worms won't have the fruit. This berry is rich in vitamin C, glucides, pectins, a trace of a certain tannic compound and considerable amounts of valuable organic acids. The mature berry has a violet-black tint due to its rare anthrocyanoside richness.

Mulberries, when available, make excellent puddings, jams, jellies and pies, as well as a medicinal syrup used to heal wounds and that is generally good for skin problems. It is mildly astringent and antibiotic. An extract of mulberry, following a thousands-of-years-old recipe, is an effective antidiarrhetic.

The mulberry is rare here. As a rule it is seen in some Italian gardens producing berries and wisely used. It is worth the effort to encourage importation of the berry and to use it in foods.

From our personal research, Caucasus peoples who have had the benefit of the mulberry as a staple in childhood tend to be without illnesses, have better than average teeth and live longer.

Mulberry leaf tisane (tea) is scarce. Mulberry's value in silkworm culture is so great that it is not likely ever to be very different. A California mulberry expert we met in Armenia told us he was attending a silk growers' conference there. At the time, he said, a top Swiss pharmaceutical firm was making strenuous efforts to buy tons of mulberry leaves, without much success. The rumor was that they were interested in an anticancer remedy using mulberry leaves. They were, our informant told us, ready to pay top prices for the leaves. In that connection, the *Vinca major*, or related "rose type"—a cousin of the pink periwinkle—has interested leading Swiss and French botanico-chemists.

A public constantly asking suppliers for mulberries would, I believe, eventually stimulate demand for this valuable natural product. Both the berries and the leaves are high on my list of valuable foods. As to priorities, I personally believe that the human order should outrank the silkworm when it comes to availability of this storehouse of natural secrets.

ONION (and the slimming group)

For centuries, large fresh-poached onions in broth, taken frequently, have been known as a reducing agent. From personal observation, I agree that the formula works.

Other reducers are fennel, particularly the lower stalks; artichoke, consumed without fattening oils or dressings; Jerusalem artichokes; and leek, cabbage, Brussels sprouts—all Spartan foods. Others, more exotic, are sea-plant products, karaya gum and chia seeds—these used to thicken soups and stews, providing bulk.

Herbal "secrets" in little-known reducers in the United States stretch from such soothing items as *maté* teas to *khat* or *Catha edulis,* once *Celastrus edulis,* which keep people at their work without cravings and without putting on weight.

This is a large subject and the uninitiate court danger by delving into it without exact knowledge and help. We mention it only to point a finger at another set of possibilities in plant life, part of a more than fanciful lore very nearly lost in antiquity. The fact is that if we will surrender the far more fanciful notion that a single pill or nostrum will save us all, it is pitifully clear that salvation lies all about us provided we accept the less palatable notion that there's work in it.

Onions, related to garlic, possess many of the same virtues. People who "hate onions" and "can't stand" garlic have a great deal of spadework to do on their attitudes if survival and longevity interest them.

SESAME

I call sesame a Caucasus youth secret. The unchemicalized seeds are great bread toppings. They are excellent in nut-cup mix with pistachios, almonds and walnuts, also Caucasus favorites. Sesame paste (tahini) has many uses, is cholesterol-free and contains iron and niacin. It is rich in unsaturated oils and supplies magnesium, 19.1 g. per 100 proteins (compare cream cheese with 8.0 g.).

Unhulled sesame seed furnishes lots of fiber; 100 g. of hulled sesame yields 2.4 g. of fiber, 110 mg. of calcium, 2.4 mg. of iron, 592 mg. of phosphorus, plus vitamins B_1, B_2 and niacin. The protein content of sesame oil compares very favorably to any other I know. Olive and corn oil offer none.

Again, space doesn't allow the kind of discussion I would like to have on sesame, but we have mentioned it in enough detail, I think, to get you started in its use in your own and your family's interest.

TAMARIND

From my own office experience, I agree that fruit pulp from this tree growing in the semitropical Caucasus, Caesalpine areas, Africa and India is useful for promoting health.

Tamarind contains pectins, some soft fiber, sugary glucides, tartaric and citric acids and a potassium compound of natural tartrate.

It is great for relieving chronic constipation. A physician colleague and I tried it on a dozen children. Their diets were the usual low-fiber type American children eat these days. On tamarind pulp, the dozen children all began immediate recovery. We tried a second dozen with equal success.

I mentioned this to a 300-pound adult male with severe chronic constipation. Even the most effective standard remedies didn't work for him. He doubted if anything that aided mere children could help him but, in desperation, he humored me. One spoonful started him back to complete normalcy. Today, with tamarind as his only medicine, he remains free of all signs and symptoms.

In the last twenty-five years, America has had the highest rate of hospitalization for G.I. problems. We have more ulcers, more diverticulitis, appendicitis, dyspepsia and colon cancer than anywhere else. We have more surgical abdomen emergencies, operations, illnesses and deaths. Tamarind is obviously worth knowing about and using correctly in avoiding much of this kind of human misery.

A story I heard from U.S. Department of Agriculture workers makes my case for herbs and botanicals. In spring, they have observed, as the mating and reproductive season nears, mink and other carnivores are seen rummaging around for botanicals, digging them up and feeding on them. Mother Nature has no billboards advertising the virtues of these plants to "lesser" creatures. But animals find their own way, generation after generation, to strengthen their reproductive apparatus and have their young through laws they obey by instinct.

Contrast this with women, especially older ones, losing baby after baby despite the refinements of modern medicine, until those fortunate enough to be put on botanicals, the kinds the carnivores grub out of the earth, suddenly find themselves able to have a live healthy baby.

Taken as a whole, food chemistry has not truly benefitted mankind. It would be incorrect to indict food processing and alteration as the chief villains of our time. They are part of a whole. We were not conditioned to survive in an atmosphere in which we inhale pollution from the air, imbibe it in our water, ingest it in our food. All of us, and especially those additionally assaulted by the environment in which they work, are standing targets for the combined effects of our total exposure to pollutants in the air, the earth, our water and our food.

Humankind is amply warned to take action against all the polluters. Meantime, we can reduce their total impact on our systems in every way open to us now by reducing the poisons in our foods, drugs, medicaments, beverages and vital water, ourselves making inroads against a rising tide in deaths from cancer and cardiovascular problems. While presidential commissions study the question and while an increasingly aware public demands health study and action, the public can lead the way by seeing to its own health through a return to natural ways.

In our brief case for herbs and botanicals, as I indicated, we have barely opened the door. We have covered the nutritional but not medicinal values, for instance, in wheat and the whole grains; we haven't gone into plantain for circulatory problems; eucalyptus leaves and their role in relieving respiratory disease and diabetes; green leaves like aloe for wound healing; natural mold preparations; the vaster range of tisanes than those barely skimmed; and special qualities and powers in vegetables and fruits.

We are indeed not powerless, although it sometimes seems that way. We need not live out our years coping with allergy, pain, breakdown, disease and their varied symptoms until premature death. Herbs and botanicals are as important a part of the solution today as they have been since primitive time. Use them for better, longer life.

7. Sex

I am aware of the deep yearning of the obese for an easy way to get thin. There's an even greater human hunger for an easy road to sexual satisfaction. These two desires, to be thin and to be satisfied sexually, have spawned thousands of books in every language.

But endless easy-weight-off books haven't cured obesity. And wisdom from all over the world on how to achieve better sexual results hasn't abated patient complaints of premature ejaculation, frigidity and every shade of failure and unhappiness in between.

Sex-book readers, I'm told, prefer explicit literature. Here, we're less interested in prurient appeal than in pointing people to a healthier, longer life, and *as a natural consequence of achieving that,* through better nutritional habits, providing the high dividend of improved sexual performance and satisfaction.

Of course, strong emotional and mental components exist in sexual inadequacy. Even so, I am satisfied that if nutritional deprivation is present or at the root of the problem, no panacea recommended will work if it doesn't include nutritional-balance restoration.

Passions can be inflamed by prurient reading or by legions of aphrodisiacs that may provide temporary results by autosuggestion or by luck. Playing new games in bed, if both parties are willing and comfortable with them, may work for a while for some. They may also provide new disappointments and setbacks. A serious side effect for some is a heart attack from trying to think young with an old body.

If any of these "solutions" really worked, we wouldn't have six hundred sex clinics in the United States today, with more opening their doors every day. And will the sex clinics, our latest fad, work? Not for anyone whose glands, directly or indirectly involved with feeding the sex organs, are nutritionally deprived!

We won't be titillating you with a new way in bed, nor even with Caucasus folklore (there's plenty) for lovemaking, greater erections and how to achieve perfectly timed mutual orgasm. Our country has imported enough written fantasies, allegedly practiced in every other part of the world. No doubt, those countries get their share of our "secrets" for achieving the same results. These "secrets" have one thing in common. Though they have provided endless hours of diversion and stimulation to the suggestible, they don't work because they change nothing, teach nothing and are scientifically without basis.

Can better sex result from natural remedies and better nutrition? I'll cite some case histories of mine, confessing I have disguised them (but in no way altered their outcomes) to spare anyone from being recognized or embarrassed.

I'll call our first case Daniel. His severe problems were not much helped by the fact that some of his relatives were doctors. Both Daniel and his wife had had the benefit of all kinds of testing before Kegan and I saw him.

At the outset of Daniel's marriage, a fine sexual relationship existed. Then something went wrong. Daniel suddenly lost his power. Both sides of the family were plunged into the battle to remedy the situation. Finally, with everyone at wits' ends, it seemed that the only way out was divorce. Psychiatry, psychology and conventional medicine had proved of no avail.

Worse than that, Daniel had been rendered a human wreck—severely depressed, demoralized, hostile, suspicious, threatening. He now refused all medicine and drugs, and was refusing to leave the house, to work, to do anything useful at all.

As often happens in these cases, someone thought of us as a last resort. Really last—we followed legal intervention, ministers and even spiritual healers.

With Daniel now promising death to anyone who even mentioned the sexual problem, Kegan and I came armed with a last-ditch remedy of our own. Keeping away from the forbidden subject, we persuaded him to look in a mirror and see how run-down he looked. "Daniel," I said, "you look terrible. Let's do something about that run-down condition and maybe you'll *feel* better."

We produced our problem-solver in a bottle. We promised that if he drank the contents we'd leave and never return.

He made a quick choice between throwing our bottle at us and drinking it to get rid of us. He did the latter, gulping it down without stopping.

We kept our word. We left immediately. Overnight, Daniel became a new man. His sexual performance returned. His amiable disposition rapidly restored, he left the house and got a job. Within a year, a beautiful, normal, full-term baby was born to him and his wife.

What magic was this? Knowing we would never get a second chance at Daniel, after considerable consultation between us Kegan brought forth from our laboratory a botanical bomb using just about everything we knew that had yielded results before.

I am professionally embarrassed to put into print one of the items in that bottle. I wouldn't use it today. Kegan's herb and botanical recipes have long since proven themselves. We don't have to resort to folk medicine today. But earlier in our practice we used more of the "medicine" handed down from generation to generation in Armenia. We combined herbals with an occasional exotic touch.

The extra ingredient was an extract compounded from a secretion of a three-day-old baby girl exhibiting a natural phenomenon known to the medical profession as "witch's milk." This not abnormal state is believed by endocrinologists to involve special hormones related to progesterone and lactogenic hormones augmented by endocrine estrogen secretions of the mother while the fetus is in the womb. The phenomenon is sometimes found at birth. The baby's breasts are enlarged and actually secrete milk.

We also recommended to Daniel a whole natural food diet for the long term to restore what was lacking in his constitution. We may have been very lucky with our nutrient cocktail, the product of desperation. But plainly, all Daniel needed was one piece of evidence that he could break out of his cocoon of impotence. Given that, he moved forward diligently. For years, family reports have bolstered our faith in what we did, though I must admit we have seldom seen results occur as fast as with Daniel.

In addition to listing the more common foods that supply our vitamins and minerals (Chapters 4 and 5), I have indicated many botanicals with the same vitamins and mineral values. Don't neglect to review them until you are familiar with all of them. Many are favorites in my laboratory for producing results in a variety of human ailments, sex problems included.

If you find it strange having a physician recommend herbs and botanicals, I am afraid I must agree that it *is* strange. Given only a conventional medical grounding, without exposure to Dr. Herbert Evans's or to Kegan's work, I might never have acquired the appreciation of a natural approach to nutrition.

Kegan had learned about nutrient values in herb and botanical extracts in use for centuries. The Evans team, myself included, had added considerable knowledge of *why* and *how* such extracts worked. Together, Kegan and I learned more. And part of what we learned applies very much to improved performance in sex.

Another instructive case history is that of Mrs. O. Married at nineteen, she was twenty-five when I first saw her, slim, shapely, very attractive—and childless. Both she and her husband had had one medical workup after another before coming to us. They had been to sex clinics. Both were in apparently perfect condition. He had a normal sperm count. They enjoyed sex, loved each other, but—no child.

Her menses were regular and normal. Her gynecological, endocrine, neurological, internal medicine, psychological and psychiatric pictures were ideal as far as examination could determine. Declared 100 percent as a potential mother, she couldn't have a child. Then there were those headaches—frequent, persistent, sometimes numbing.

The couple had been advised to have more frequent sex, then less frequent sex. They had been schooled in sex positioning, in the gentle art of sex foreplay, had read everything on sex, diet, health and whatever else was suggested. They were so well-schooled that if they wanted to, they could operate a sex clinic today. But no baby, and those headaches persisted.

A family member told us about her. We insisted there be no buildup, no promises that we could help. We told her on our first meeting that barrenness is no crime; that some of the world's loveliest ladies, including royal queens, had been able to enjoy sex without reproducing.

Leading her to expect nothing, we prescribed a regimen of herbs and botanical extracts despite the absence of outward signs of ill health. She soon found the headaches loosening their grip and, though beautiful before, she truly began to blossom. She saw the difference as people began regularly complimenting her appearance. Within three months she missed her period, rushed to the obstetrician and was shortly declared pregnant.

She had a beautiful baby who should now be in early grade school. We have kept up through her family and hear she's fine. She has come over, as most of our patients have, to whole natural foods, abandoning fanatically processed, chemicalized junk foods heavily constituted of refined white sugar and refined white flour.

I have treated men getting on in years, not worried about inability to produce offspring but simply hating to slow down sexually, wanting to feel "more like men" again. Most men hate turning into sexual neuters. Habit alone makes continuation of sexual ability a barometer for health and state of mind.

Many of these older male patients know some or all the standard remedies—zinc tablets, weight control, fresh green vegetables, yeast, multivitamins and minerals. When we add a range of botanical extracts that administer extra amounts of good-tasting vitamins and minerals directly from nature, we seem to get extraordinarily good results. Some of those results are:

- Deeper, more pleasant, more manly voices
- Improved strength and endurance for sex and general purposes
- Maintained or improved hair color
- End to slowdown; better job performance
- End to insomnia, complained of by many

This last should not surprise anyone. Dwindling sexual ability, life's strains and poor nutrition are an excellent route to chronic insomnia. As indicated, I have cured many such problems.

Mr. X and Mr. Y, both older men who joke today about near brushes with death and both solidly indoctrinated in our total health for longevity plan, each individually vow that they will break 100. I mention these two because they were among the worst prospects I have treated. Now, a number of years into our regimen, I see no reason why both shouldn't make 100 or more if they keep at it, stay with our dietary suggestions (I doubt if either will ever go back to the old junk food), and continue getting regular help from botanical extracts and herbs in their salads and soups. Footnote: One of these men, crowding sixty, has resumed an active sex life.

There are all kinds of sex-related difficulties, some self-induced. For instance, nothing discourages attractiveness to a partner more than foul odors, from the mouth or anywhere else. I know this subject is less than pleasant, but let's just get at it.

Some human odors are attractive, some are not. I have had patients with mouth odors caused by defective teeth and gums, nasal or throat conditions giving chronic offense and stomach odors or ear discharges keeping mates at bay. Running sores, internal or on the skin, call for referral and clearing up, usually followed by resumption of better sexual relations. Those are simple items. When such conditions are cleared and sex problems persist, usually a botanical extract will make the difference.

A case in point—Miss V. Nobody could tell her at work, but her vegetarian diet caused a chronic foul stool odor that others found obnoxious. When she came to me, she was on the point of leaving her well-paid job. She told me she had overheard her co-workers discussing her problem (and theirs). I convinced her that if she left she would only take the problem with her to a new environment unless we did something to change things. And if we did change things, she could stay on her present job.

She saw logic in that and held her job as we experimented with wholesome extracts, entirely consistent with her vegetarianism, adding fiber and other nutrients that altered her intestinal effluents. The problem disappeared. She made friends with her staff without a word ever being spoken about the former offense.

We have similarly helped others with allergies, with sharp loss in sense of smell, loss of taste sensation, with chronically coated tongues and with other conditions uniquely contributing to loss of ability to participate in rewarding sex experiences, to hostility and resentment, to frigidity or impotence.

I would like to offer this observation on the subject. Sense of smell is part of the mysticism of sex itself. Though many men find the normal odor at the vagina attractive, many women are ashamed of it. Such an attitude among women is the result of conditioning, and a few written words can't change that overnight. But women who keep themselves normally clean needn't really be concerned about their husbands' reactions. Any man himself not conditioned to think of sex as dirty and vaginal odors part of that will find her attractive totally and very likely will be stimulated, not repelled, by everything about her vagina.

In saying that I don't place too much faith in new experiments in sex to improve performance, I must also state that I believe two consenting adults, comfortable enough with each other to experiment, should not be inhibited by outmoded attitudes handed on by their rather stifled antecedents.

In the same personal habits vein, too many women use excess perfumes and toiletries, often in clashing combinations, either to disguise body odors or to cast, they think, an aura of attractiveness. Most men like their woman to have a subtle fragrance, one they come to identify with her. But if women are blotting pads for every new scent on the market, that's overkill. And women who use scents to disguise body odors usually fool nobody. Scents and body odors can be nauseating combinations, repellents.

For men and women both, regular soap and water washing and neat grooming are fine sex aids. If soap and water is against your religion (it is in some parts of the world), marry within your religion!

If you're in normal health and without the problems mentioned above (or problems as bad), you can avoid offending after onions or garlic by chewing on mint leaves or parsley. It's also wise with cabbage, onions or garlic to share those foods with your mate. If both indulge, neither offends.

People who are allergy-prone can avoid mouth odors (and usually other discomforts) by using salt-water rinses often, brushing teeth with a little salt instead of sweet pastes, seeing their dentists if trouble persists, avoiding alcohol, not smoking and avoiding meat or any foods that produce allergic reactions and often odors at the mouth.

I am not unique in seeing the joy of sex more in terms of what a couple wants mutually (for each other as well as for self) out of marriage, and less in terms of length of time before orgasm or frequency of intercourse. Partners who make the grade are less interested in keeping score than in giving and sharing. Partners not making the grade usually count, total up grievances and look for faults in their mates. Sexual failure is usually part of the failure of the overall relationship. Where this is true, I doubt if sex remedies —even sex remedies in a framework of improved nutrition—will do much good.

Primeval man, in the Caucasus and elsewhere, was characterized by a taste for mating and sex durability. Man's primitive instincts led him to sex-and-survival foods. We know this from Neolithic drawings, cave relics (many in Armenia and Azerbaijan), archeological digs and ancient inscriptions elsewhere.

Animal-protein foods were strongly favored from the beginning. But not only *animal* proteins—a hybrid wheat appeared first in Armenia after the Ice Age. This was crossed with goat's wheat, developed to later hybrid forms, moved across Europe and eventually arrived here as baker's wheat.

For centuries and centuries Caucasus people have favored raw milk, starting children with one year's breast feeding, continuing them on fermented milks (yogurt, *kefir*) and gradually adding nearly every item in the menu—soups, appetizers, salads, main courses and desserts.

These were among the earliest peoples to tame animals for transportation and for food. Discovering milk, they were quick to use it as a food, in other foods, in cooking, in yogurt and then preserved as cheese. Even the whey wasn't wasted.

They learned early to rely on the protein in eggs, every kind from birds' to fish roe. Omelets, eggs with spinach and eggs with greens filled in nicely when meat supplies grew low. Habits cling. Game bird eggs are still delicacies in the Caucasus.

Earlier we mentioned certain foods believed in the Caucasus to help afford better sexual performance. Remember the common belief among Armenian oldsters to this day that lamb's testicles make the perfect sex food? *Of course* there's something to it. I call such foods source foods, fundamental foods. And I include with testicles of every edible animal all the vital organ foods, reservoirs of the body's nutritional needs. I further include all edible seeds, for such seeds are power-packed with entire nutritional complexes for the generation of new life. Wheat is seed, sesame is seed, nuts are seeds and so are apple, pear, orange and apricot seeds, prune pits (you probably don't know that date pits are pounded to pieces and given to camels), pumpkin seeds, sunflower seeds, watermelon seeds, canteloupe and melon seeds.

Remember my telling you that people pour vitamins and minerals away with the vegetable cooking water? They do as badly throwing away the seeds of apples, pears and the rest. Pressed from their pods, pounded or chewed out, these small storehouses nature gave the ability to create new generations, are valuable dietary additions with sexual benefits. Pound the prune pits. Add the seeds to your cooking and baking. Get those small bits and pieces of nutrition you've been casually discarding for years. Enjoy them, enjoy finding them as cost-free add-ons to your diet, not only for economy (reason enough) but for the knowledge that they provide vital extras in nutrition enrichment.

Similarly, save the skins of fruits. Eat them. Remember, in the growing process they took in the sunlight, vitamin D and other atmosphere-borne benefits.

I am not suggesting that we turn away from balanced foods and concentrate on these source foods. A little at any one meal goes a long way. But don't neglect this ready wealth in energy source foods, yours with every purchase of fruits, nuts, meats, poultry, fish, whole wheat, seeds, grains and so on endlessly. For many, this thinking must replace attitudes and conditioning of a lifetime. But the battle for longer life, better health and improved sex performance very likely requires most of us to examine and change habits and attitudes of a lifetime. Nobody said it would be simple. But I tell you it can be done. I see it happening in my practice. I read of it happening in case histories written up by colleagues. And I saw evidence of it in the Caucasus where sex at 100 is common and sex at 120 is not as uncommon as one might believe.

Now let's get down to what I'm calling my Big Twelve foods for improved sexual performance. (You can prepare them from recipes in our recipe section.) The first is Barbara Apisson's own delicious soup, a West Point Farms favorite for many years, enjoyed by a clientele that for the most part don't know its secret ingredient.

The soup, *pahrtabour*, has had overwhelming acceptance because it tastes wonderful. Barbara and Henri, from the beginning, have never told patrons about that one ingredient (you'll learn it in the recipe section), correctly afraid that Americans would refuse to try it, depriving themselves of its great source-food benefits. For the same reason, such items as blackstrap molasses disappeared years ago from West Point Farms tables. But Barbara continues her culinary magic in the kitchen, out of sight of patrons who reap great rewards without knowing why.

I put *pahrtabour* first on my Big Twelve sex-nutrients list, which follows shortly. Other items, which should be eaten regularly to restore what bodies may lack for better sexual performance, include dishes prepared with liver, heart, meat-and-kidney mixtures, sweetbreads, homemade sausage-type dishes, spleen, the use of marrow as a spread or in soups (marrow, my vegetarian friends, is a storehouse of bone building blocks). And all these dishes in variations are made more palatable and adventurous with pungent herbs, health-giving botanicals and delicate spices.

I do sympathize with those whose life-styles make at least some of the above an acceptance problem. ("I *hate* vegetables." "Liver? *Me* eat liver?" "Spleen?" "*Sweet*breads?") But here we are at war with common sense. Are you below par nutritionally? Is your sex life less than it should be? Are you one of the millions in America headed for a life expectancy of 65, or 55 or less when it could be 75 and 85 or 100 or more? Don't tell me about what you will or won't eat! This book is all about *changing* your habits, lengthening your life, making you feel better as you live longer. Get with it! Please, no closed minds. Shake off your prejudices. Open your thinking to new and what I promise will be only temporarily strange tastes. By ridding yourself of body-killing habits and trying out something new, you'll be no different from my patients, who were dismayed at first thought but desperate enough with their aches and illnesses to decide they had nothing to lose by trying.

My patients have in this way won new zest for living, new bodies, more years and improved sexual performance and enjoyment. Don't doubt us. Join us. You have only yourself to help.

The meatless proteins we need come in cheeses, yogurt, *plaki* (baked) with beans, fish *plaki,* whole grains, whole wheat, lentils, millet, soybeans and vegetables. All these are common sources of meatless protein in the Caucasus. A variety of preparation techniques (see our recipe section) fancy them up so that nobody misses the meat.

Our next chapter is on exercise. You can't enjoy total sexual pleasure with a chronically inactive body. But let's save that for Chapter 8 and enumerate now what I call the Big Twelve foods for sexual balance. I'll comment on a number of them. What I'm suggesting is that, to improve your sexual performance, emphasis on the Big Twelve in your diet will help measurably to phenomenally.

The Big Twelve

1. *Pahrtabour* soup
2. *Petmez*
3. *Tahini*
4. Eggs, roe, *tarama*
5. Whole-wheat group
6. Yogurt group
7. Specialty organ meats, liver, fish-liver oils
8. Snails, mussels, shellfish, fish, dulse, kelp
9. Greens and the big yellow vegetables
10. Fruits, nuts, seeds, grains, beans
11. Herbs, botanicals
12. Miscellaneous (supplements)

Does the schooled reader quickly detect that honey is missing? That's no accident. I've read every honey bible and decided that the claims for honey actually apply to pollen in unrefined honey, dark natural honey, the only kind to eat, sparingly. But since obesity and sex fall-off go hand in chubby hand, the smart sex dieter must avoid honey as he or she does any sugar, instead buying the pollen in health-food stores or by mail order. Pollen is another of nature's storehouses for a new generation of living matter and is, I believe, a worthwhile nutrient for mankind. (However, if you are addicted to sweets and can't break away, I'd rather you had dark honey than refined white sugar products which are empty of nutrients.)

Let's run down some of our Big Twelve. Why, you might ask, turn to something foreign for sex nutrition? Well, if you've already shopped around and the eggs, oysters, brandy-nogs, mandrake roots, ginseng and such haven't done it for you, is this a time to Buy American or to try something new that may help you?

A chunk of organ meat Barbara Apisson uses in *pahrtabour* soup (roughly 5″ x 2½″ in size), ground up so finely that you have no idea what you're eating except that it tastes very good, is shown to contain 3.4 percent of your RDA of calories; 25 percent protein, 3 percent fat, 714 percent niacin, 8 percent sodium, 9 percent phosphorus and 7 percent iron. All this, as a rule, from an organ of a frisky male calf. This protein source is glandular, yet gelatinizes beautifully and digests as well.

People who dislike eggs, shellfish, seaweed, beef, lamb, liver, heart, brain and the like will not only love *pahrtabour*, they *need* it. Incidentally, the French dote on this particular protein, known for its ability (via its surface cells) to elaborate enzymes. Tests show it helps the anemic. Extracts of its deeper substance produce another protein that helps people lose weight.

I am convinced that *pahrtabour* gives good building blocks and high support to our amino acids. People who have *pahrtabour* soup regularly look younger than their years. Isn't that worth turning to something new and foreign for?

Number two on our Big Twelve list for better sex nutrition is *petmez.* Native to the area bounded by the Black and Caspian seas, we have mentioned this naturally concentrated grape extract a number of times. Under various spellings and variants, *petmez* can be found in specialty import groceries, particularly those of the Syrians, Greeks, Italians, Armenians and Lebanese.

Naturally, I hope this book stimulates greater import of *petmez.* Describe it to your grocer and keep after him to have his supplier run it down for you. It's worth this effort.

Many who teach nutrition say that no fruit except the apple in a minor role helps us achieve sex-performance balance. I point to *petmez,* containing grape concentrate of rich mineral origin. Raw grapes digest in under two hours. As *petmez* extract, the product digests even faster.

Twenty-four medium-sized European grapes, approximating a generous serving of *petmez* on bread or in cookery, provide 2.5 percent of our RDA in calories; .9 percent protein; 5.8 percent carbohydrate; .5 percent fat, or unsaturated oil; 3.8 percent vitamin B_1, or thiamine; 3.6 percent B_2, or riboflavin; 1.6 percent niacin; 2 percent vitamin A; 6 percent potassium; 3 to 4 percent iron; considerable chromium and sulfur compounds, very important to us; plus vitamin C and other mineral traces.

European sanitoriums have long appreciated the therapeutic value of grapes. Their potassium tartrate helps stimulate urine flow, washing out body poisons and aiding the kidneys. Grapes stimulate healthy perspiration, alkalize the system and act as a laxative to some people or regulators of the intestinal tract.

Caucasus people smile when someone mentions *petmez.* It's a joy-giver, used in many ways in their cuisine—for instance, in combination with *tahini* (sesame paste), which is also available in specialty import groceries. When you find *petmez,* stock up on it. It gives out quickly and time slips by between shipments.

If all Americans knew *petmez* from birth instead of refined white sugar, with our high level of medical advances *we'd* be in better shape sexually, generally, and live longer, healthier lives than people do now in the Caucasus.

Number three on our Big Twelve list is *tahini,* sesame paste, which you might call Armenian peanut butter. Peanuts grow there, but the preference for *tahini* is so great that you see little peanut butter.

Sesame is described as containing a hormonal-type building block. I have seen claims that it contains traces of compounds related to testosterone and progesterone. No special powers are credited to sesame paste in the United States, and it has little popularity here outside of certain ethnic minorities in spite of its delicious flavor and ease of use.

Get into *tahini.* The paste equivalent of one ½ cup of sesame seed provides about 23 percent of the RDA in calories, 28 percent protein, and essential amino acids as follows: 62 percent of valuable tryptophane; almost 72 percent leucine; 34 percent lysine, an amino acid the government says should be added to breads and cereals; 27 percent methionine; almost 64 percent phenylalanine; nearly 54 percent isoleucine, 52 percent valine; 67 percent threonine; 95.3 percent fat, much of this unsaturated and rich in vitamins E and F; 5 to 6 percent carbohydrate; 13.9 percent B_1; 7.9 percent B_2; 29.4 percent niacin; 49 percent phosphorus; 14 percent calcium; 21 percent iron. Depending on seed type, from 40 to 55 percent is reported as oil. Sesame is also high in choline and inositol, lecithin components and lecithin itself, a major constituent of human semen and important to nerve and brain tissues. The master gland, the pituitary, and the pineal gland—both keystones in sex performance—contain greater lecithin concentrations than any other parts of the body. Other *tahini* values are magnesium, sulfur and potasium.

Since Babylonian times, women have treasured sesame seeds, using sesame paste and honey (*halvah*) to restore male virility. While I believe refined honey doesn't provide pollen as those ancient concoctions did, sesame paste is, as you've seen, a treasure trove of nutrients many agree are helpful in sexual performance.

Among Middle Easterners (especially Armenians), *tahini,* called *matahini,* is noted as a sexual-therapeutic agent, rejuvenator of physical capacity, restorer of stamina and sexual endurance. Cultivated for thousands of years, it's mentioned frequently in ancient writings as a powerful sex food. Its composition shows us why this is so.

Number four on our Big Twelve list, roe, *tarama* and other forms of eggs, enjoy an equally long history as credited sex foods. Roe is the leading choice in many countries besides the Caucasus.

As chicken eggs do, roe furnishes considerable thiamine, riboflavin and pantothenate; is protein-rich, particularly in high-quality tryptophane, leucine, isoleucine, methionine, phenylalanine, lysine, valine and threonine; and contains vitamins A, D, E and F, some lecithin and cholesterol, plus iron, copper, phosphorus, chromium, a good deal of zinc and sometimes a trace of hormone. As distinct from eggs whose shells contain the calcium, roe offers more than a trace of calcium. Roe is richer, too, in iodide and fluoride than animal eggs whose donors may be deficient, diet-wise, in the nutritional riches available in seawater and sea plants.

Emphasizing again, roe, like sesame seeds, raw nuts, beans, fish livers, whole grains and other source foods, directly or less directly serving a species as "eggs" for reproductive purposes, has drawn peoples for hundreds of centuries as a sex food. And this fascination is far from nonsense.

Recent tests bear out the value of these foods. Using as a criterion unhampered growth, these tests showed that egg is a food animals can grow up on, reproduce on, live on and prosper on as long as they can on a good mixed diet. Egg is the only material thus far of which this has been found to be true. As good as many other foods are, they do not singly support growth and development as eggs do, even when unsupplemented. Think that over.

And so we see these tests vindicating the great respect seen in the Caucasus for *tarama,* sturgeon roe, for enhancement of amatory powers and sexual endurance.

I cannot speak well of dried eggs, often stale at that, imported into this country in drums for use in processed commercial foods and by larger bakeries.

Number five on our Big Twelve list for better sex is the whole-wheat group. Here I do not mean wheat-germ oil or even the isolated germ of wheat by itself, but good whole grains, parts not separated.

Historians disagree as to whether wheat or rice was first cultivated in the Caucasus. Whichever, according to Neolithic evidence man found wheat the easier to cultivate, harvest, store and transport.

Wheat is the only grain with high-gluten protein (rye has a little), responsible for leavening. For lightness or rising, wheat breadstuffs are better than those made of grains, seeds, beans or rice.

Wheat protein is not equal to soybean protein, but whole-wheat bread can be eaten with soybeans or any beans for balance, and wheat products go nicely with any course, from soup through dessert.

Where are the sexual benefits? Besides containing vitamin E, which preserves well if the germ is not separated, wheat is rich in vitamin F. One cup of whole fresh wheat contains on the average about 16 percent of the RDA in calories and 24 percent in protein. Processed wheat made into white flour is short on lysine and loses much of its vitamin E, chromium, selenium and zinc—all important sex nutrients.

That same cupful of unprocessed natural high-quality whole wheat has the following percentages of RDAs of these valuable protein constituents: 38.4 percent tryptophane; 48.7 percent leucine; 49.1 percent isoleucine; 46 percent valine; 46.4 percent threonine; 27 percent lysine; 35.6 percent phenylalanine and 11.8 percent methionine. Other RDA factors are 25.1 percent carbohydrate; 4.3 percent fat, as wheat-germ oil; 53.9 percent B_1; 8.1 percent B_2; 27.3 percent niacin; 7.1 percent vitamin B_6, or pantothenate, important for a healthy pituitary gland; and 16 percent pantothenic acid. Other RDA constituents of wheat are 33 percent folic acid; 3 percent B_{12}; 24.4 percent choline; a considerable amount of inositol; and, as indicated, vitamins E and F. Minerals found in wheat include chromium, zinc, phosphorus, iron, calcium, copper, magnesium and potassium. All wheat also has some manganese, although buckwheat is richer in this essential.

As Dr. Evans and his group discovered in the earlier work at Berkeley, two tablespoons of fresh wheat germ give 1 g. of linoleic acid, a high yield of vitamin E and all the components mentioned above.

Please scan this wheat list again and then tell me why you think white bread should remain popular for your health and your family's.

Number six on our Big Twelve list is the yogurt group. Do you remember just how many vital nutrients showed up in yogurt in our Chapters 4 and 5 listings? If not, read those chapters again. And see, too, how often organ meats, led by liver, appear as vitamin and mineral sources, and how fish-liver oils and all animal and vegetable seafoods—numbers seven and eight in our Big Twelve—are rich vitamin-D sources, vital for thyroid function, which is important to sex performance.

While you're back in those chapters, read again about vegetables, fruits, nuts, seeds, beans and whole grains—numbers nine and ten on our Big Twelve list. These source foods are important to good sex function. Number eleven on our Big Twelve list, herbs and botanicals, was covered in Chapter 6.

That leaves number twelve, miscellaneous. You may need to add some other items based on what seems to work for you as an individual, but my basic number twelve is supplementation. I hope you remember and refer often to the Chapter 5 chart, which lists recommended supplementation for average adult need. As I've said, what promotes overall health promotes better sexual ability. My feeling is that readers who count poor sexual performance among their ills will be doubly helped by the supplementation suggested in the chart.

Sex is so vital a part of normal living that rewarding experience in it seems little enough to ask of life. For many of us, improved diet will provide the key to healthy organs and orgasms. Serious attention to our Big Twelve list and to all the dietary data you'll find in Chapters 10 and 11 will show you the way, just as our suggestions on exercise for fitness, in the next chapter, will play their part.

8.

Make Your Body Work by Walking and Gardening

First, people should *not* exercise vigorously if they have serious heart and vascular problems: blockages of any main coronary artery; irregular heartbeats which *doctors* have diagnosed as arrhythmia (not self-diagnosed flutters, bleeps or gurgles); severe angina pectoris; heart-valve diseases; severe high blood pressure; or any heart condition doctors describe as serious. People with such conditions must not perform any exercises not approved by their own physicians. That goes for diabetics, anemia cases and sufferers from varicose veins, too.

We would hope doctors and these patients can agree on lecithin, vitamin C and minerals such as chromium (Chapters 4 and 5) as stabilizers and improvers in these conditions. After there has been good improvement, exercise can be discussed with your doctor.

People in reasonably good health should borrow two Caucasus habits: their survivor diet and physical labor as a way of life.

Kegan and I saw in the Caucasus the daily demands made on young and old bodies alike. True, we can't build mountains where there are none. But most of us can get to hills and stairs and take walks instead of buses, subways, taxicabs and cars.

There are exercises even for the handicapped. Believe me, flexing and unflexing muscles, clenching and unclenching fists is useful work. Clenching and unclenching toes, deep knee bends, trunk exercises, bending and straightening legs and arms, any calisthenics that are possible, practiced daily *on a gradually rising routine*, are ways of warding off atrophy of body, mind and enthusiasm. For all but the totally limbless or paralyzed, there is something.

Between you and your doctor, if you are two-legged and two-armed, with normal ability to make your body work, you can get into motion, slowly at first, and gradually increase your exercises, stretching your maximum a bit at a time, until you have built a body best able to benefit from improved nutrition.

Why should *you* get up off your martini-side perch and rediscover exercise? Without getting highly technical, I can assure you that people persuaded to exercise after habitual sedentary lives prove to have better working hearts, better oxygen utility by their systems, greater stamina and better general health afterwards than before. Just as important, a rising program of exercise reduces weight even if diet remains the same as before, and works to tone up the muscles generally.

These words or *something* (such as the desire to live longer) must first motivate you to exercise. You've got to want to change yourself for the better to get started. You do that much, and exercise plus our diet will do wonders for you, naturally and without risk.

I do not recommend, in fact I heartily discourage, weekend athletics. If you're deskbound five days a week, don't fan out over the tennis courts, handball courts, golf courses (especially when the sun is high, hot and punishing) for one or two intense days a weekend. Those irregular bursts of energy don't do you the good you may think. Also, they can be dangerous. I've seen too many weekend athletes in emergency wards, still in sports clothes, gasping for breath.

I'm not suggesting you *stop* your sports. If you enjoy them, by all means schedule a moderate amount on the weekend. But don't lean on these alone as your salute to exercise. Build around these weekends other forms of exercise during the week. For health and longevity, make body work a seven-day-a-week proposition and *gradually* add minutes and hours of daily exercise until you have given yourself back what your own efforts to succeed in sedentary endeavors have taken away. Let's see an end to the stream of forty-year-old executives dying at their desks or on commuter trains between inactivities.

No time for this? Nonsense. By making your body work as I suggest, you are creating extra years of time to be successful, enjoy family life, enjoy recreation and really enjoy the zest of being alive once you free your body from nonphysical existence.

Looking at it the other way, lack of work and lack of opportunity for your legs and organs to respirate through effort will positively deprive you of years you can gainfully and joyously use. Think of our process, you hard-driven success freaks, as investment for gain. Share with your tension-making business activity a rising regimen of tension-breaking body work for extra years to enjoy the fruits of success and be glad you're alive.

If you make no time for this foolishness, you can't help yourself a bit. But if you have an open mind and desire to keep or restore your vigor, there's no end to what you can accomplish in the battle for survival.

Time for the perfect example, Harry S Truman! I have all the facts on his remarkable case from Dr. George S. Carter. I wrote Dr. Carter's biography from personal interviews and from correspondence with his famous patient. President Truman attributed his health, pep and longevity to his physician.

Mr. Truman had been a weak-legged, prematurely aging U.S. Senator. The change began as he saw his colleagues in the Congress dropping around him. A man of more than normal courage, he couldn't help being affected by so many premature deaths. He asked Dr. Carter, "Will I be next?"

Dr. Carter pulled no punches. "I don't know how you've lasted this long with your unused body. From haberdashery to politics, living in smoke-filled rooms until you reached the Senate, Mr. Truman, you're in worse shape right now than some of your colleagues who are dead."

Dr. Carter told me, "I just laid it on the line. Walk or die! No options. Senator Truman promised to try if I could help get him started."

The doctor put Mr. Truman on mild leg exercises in the beginning, a routine to build up his leg muscles for the walking to come. Then he began short leisurely walks to get the leg muscles to come alive, to strengthen gradually.

Continually, Dr. Carter checked heart and lungs—and diet. Senator Truman had to take off some weight and shift weight from the abdomen to the muscles and bones. He strengthened his limbs by gradually adding to the physical tax on them, avoiding any sudden activity increase that might have killed him at the outset. Slowly, Mr. Truman increased his vital capacity (heart–lung functioning) and before long the slightest effort no longer took his breath away.

We all know where it led. Harry S Truman became a legendary President. Without this effort, he might not have been alive to take his place in history in the crisis of President Roosevelt's sudden death. But he lived to outpace every reporter in Washington, New York and other cities on his early morning walks, despite the tradition that the reporter is the legman!

Mr. Truman proved you don't need mountains or hills to have a daily routine of brisk physical exercise, only brains and determination. The unhappy fact is that few politicians or businessmen can keep up with Mr. Truman's pace at the top of his form, even though their lives depend on it.

You can change your pace and prospects. You can do what Mr. Truman did. See your doctor and get started. Get to bed earlier and up earlier. Create the time for early morning walks. Begin!

One of my patients—I'll call him Nick—didn't come to me to be built up but for his routine physical. He had loved sports since childhood. He and his brothers, all hefty, healthy men, grew up on wholesome old-fashioned foods, containing no additives or chemicals. All were strong, well able in boyhood to defend themselves in New York City's downtown cauldron of ethnic disparates.

At the peak of a championship career, Nick entered the army and helped train others in manly activities usually neglected by city-slicker types in our country. After the war, he went into business for himself and eventually operated his own successful advertising agency. His work never stopped him from walking miles every day, putting in regular hours at the gym and bowling nearly nightly.

Heavy in bone and body, he benefitted from getting into our health-power dietary suggestions, trimming and improving his stamina. He lives a full life and helps others live full lives. One of his sons has become manager of a major-league baseball team. Like Harry Truman, Nick's an excellent example of what you can do with the will to keep or make yourself healthy.

Compare the sedentary lives most of us live with a scene I recall in Erivan, Armenia's capital. It was in the children's park in the heart of the city. In good weather, a ballet class does its practicing outdoors there. The girls dress in tutus, not leotards. For serious students, coaches watch timing and correctness of movements. As children reach new stages in physical growth and ability, they are allowed to move up to higher-level bodily demands. There is time only for dance and walking about and instructions, not for talking or sitting about. During one break, the future ballerinas sip a cup of orange juice.

There are child musicians under the trees. They sway with their playing. Younger children at the sidelines mimic the students, some very gracefully. Many, slated for later formal training, simply watch and imitate now.

Children under three are still chubby, in keeping with the theory of developing a strong pelvis as a foundation. This is a good general practice, not just for ballerinas but for healthy life.

After three, with the proper pelvic foundation established,

weight watching is the rule. Children selected for ballet training are trimmed to ideal slenderness.

Also at the sidelines in the children's park are the inevitable oldsters. Sometimes there are four generations on the scene. They escort the children to the park, hold their schoolbooks and bags, applaud vigorously, stamp about, some adding their own interpretations of the dancing when the spirit moves them. For all ages, the scene is one of vigor, enthusiasm, participation. Ingrained zest for movement, for body work, takes place with little thought or planning. It's natural.

Compare such a scene with the states of vegetation among the older generations of our society. With only imagination and will as limits, what a crime inactivity is against aging limbs and organs and against the very quality of living.

Primal man was concerned not only with survival but with teaching his offspring lessons of survival he had learned. So he sketched out rough cave wall pictures of animals to be feared and avoided and sketches of which forage plants had proved edible and which should be avoided.

It was uncomplicated then. Enough food had to be provided before the ravages of weather confined the group to the cave. Survival was a year-by-year contest; it was a total preoccupation—living meant tough physical struggle all the time. With careful planning, struggle could yield upwards of twenty hard years to the strong, the alert, the quick. A fortunate few outlived the form charts by a good margin.

That's our heritage. It's in our cells, our genes. With all we have learned since the first cave scratchings, pushing our average life expectancy above three score, most of us have lost sight of primal survival fundamentals that still guide those between the Black and Caspian seas as high as five score and ten, six score and more.

We can all learn from the children's park scene in Erivan and from the cave scratchings of ancient times. Both tell us the same thing—that fitness, food and fun go together for health and longevity. If longer life and better health are your goals, ignore none of the three.

I treated a fine singer. His dream had been to appear on the stage, in television, in films. He had the talent, studied prodigiously and worked with awesome dedication, but stardom never came. His diet was far from ideal and as for exercise, nil! He did find an outlet for his talent—recordings. But handicaps in weight and in a body lacking eye appeal frustrated his ambition to appear before audiences. Nutritionally and physically he was only part of what he might have been. His career, too, was only part of what it might have been.

Another case worth recalling involved a youthful American athlete I'll call Paul. He was ambitious to succeed as a skater in the Olympics. He practiced with burning zeal, skipped meals to skate and ate sparingly but not sensibly in his zeal to keep his weight down. He began his climb, taking prize after prize, but he never made the Olympics. Though his muscles were well-toned and strong, his bones lacked fundamental development.

A relatively minor fall fractured both bones of one leg. Not to be denied, Paul tried desperately to regain lost momentum, yet had another spill and another fracture. He knew this one was the end. Today he coaches younger skaters. Too late for his own ambitions, he eats more sensibly and does all he can to convince his students to do the same.

I've already said that there must be motivation, *desire* on your part, a strong stimulus right up out of your vital life force, before you'll really do anything about all this. But I am convinced you can find that motivation if you'll try. It was handed on to you as a precious gift from our common ancestors who knew what struggle meant to survival.

The gains must be worth the effort. If you aren't moved by our words, your doctor's, or your family's to be what you can be physically and nutritionally, to make yourself healthier and live longer, you may need something else before you embrace our regimen. You may need to come to terms with yourself mentally and emotionally.

We all pay a toll for our intense competitive existence. But those lively oldsters we saw in the Caucasus are spectacularly unencumbered by the complexities of our hectic and ever more difficult way of life. I do not urge scrapping our system for theirs, but putting it plainly, I think properly nourished bones take priority over bank accounts, general health priority over success. We must keep a balance to survive.

Most of us are not professional athletes. Our conditioning must be more like Mr. Truman's than Joe Namath's. So we must walk . . . walk or die. Walk every day. Walk a bit more every day. Develop a route safe from traffic, safe from running children, safe from muggers, with natural stopping points along the way if (in the begining) you tire—a friend to talk to, a bench to sit on, a store window to stare into—whatever helps you break in gradually.

Is that cab necessary? Leave earlier and walk, or walk part way and then take a bus or cab. Walk one stop, then two, then three. And so on. Do you have a car and chauffeur? Let him follow you a few blocks and then pick you up as you begin to tire. Then have him meet you at designated points, each more distant than before as time goes on. Don't let wheels deprive you of body-building walking. When the habit takes hold, see how reluctant you get to board a bus or descend into a subway.

Now let's talk about gardening. Walking and gardening are what I'd like to see you get into. I worry about many of my jogger patients for the same reason that I worry about weekend athletes. I hate to see them at the end of their jogs, color uneven, struggling for breath, near collapse. Walking to where you do your gardening is safer. You'll have items to carry to the garden; later, as they grow, you'll have items to bring from the garden. Someone you know somewhere has a piece of ground you can cultivate. Plan it. Do it.

You might get into gardening gradually, on your own patio, in your own apartment, on your windowsills in plant boxes, adding to what you start with as results make you more ambitious.

Why gardening? All over the world, people who garden tend to live longer. Vermonters, oldsters in many places where surburbanites are lucky enough to find them available to garden for them, magnificent elderly Italians and other transplants from overseas are still found travelling long distances, often on foot, to get to their own gardens or yours. And growing numbers of ordinary people, especially today's young, are driven by rising prices and idealism to stake out garden patches and do their thing. Whatever they're raising from the ground, they're benefitting their bodies with the exercise if they're doing it seriously.

Grow flowers if that's what your heart desires. I strongly recommend herbs and botanicals. As you get to know them better, you'll be glad to have your own fresh supplies of this health-giving group. I'd start with those easiest to grow but healthy to have, like mint, basil and parsley.

If you know someone in a garden club, arrange to visit. Play your spades right and maybe you'll be invited to join. I'd be willing to bet, sight unseen, that club gardeners raising and using fresh botanicals and greens are healthier than you are.

Lots of universities have associations with garden clubs. Perhaps you can come by a lecturer to get you started. Or take an extension course. One thing about gardening, you can set your own pace and choose your own crops. Gardening exercises the whole body when you do all your work from start to finish. Gardening and walking complement each other. Both build better bodies by making our bodies work. Do two exercises, not just one, but whether you try our combination or another you and your doctor concoct, get started.

There are other types of exercise, of course. There is dancing, swimming, calisthenics, horseback riding, horseshoes, light tennis, track, trapeze—name your own. But get started!

Time for a story. A professor friend of mine invited me to a meal some years ago. It was marvellous. Soup, salad, vegetable dishes, main course, dessert—everything was strange, delicious and unrecognizable. I kept prodding my host. What's this dish? What's that? Not until the dinner was over did he reveal that I had been treated to mushrooms—nothing but mushrooms found on a club outing, one variety after another, each course so cleverly prepared, so fenced about with imaginative touches, that I had no idea at any point that I was being feted with mushrooms, mushrooms and mushrooms again, twenty-seven varieties in all, all nutritious, mineral-rich, wholesome, tasty.

You can't grow mushrooms in an apartment. It takes a damp cellar. If you have one, send for the kit with complete instructions.

Probably nobody has to warn you about poisonous wild mushrooms. If you're not an absolute expert, don't pick them on outings. It's safest to get the kit, follow instructions to the letter and grow them in a damp cellar.

A group of New York City professors, students, businessmen and women, including some wealthy people, meet, ride and walk to their hobby, mushroom hunting. They are experts. They gather hundreds of edible varieties, mushrooms, truffles, related species. Mushrooms grow everywhere except in deserts. If there is a club near you, join it. Or else form one around an expert if you can find one. Mushroom hunting is a grand way to build better bodies.

But it takes a garden to grow comfrey, purslane and lamb's-quarters, contributing to healthy teas, soups, salads and entrées. They go with seafood and fish, with stews as extenders, and are both decorative and nutritious.

If you open for business in a few window boxes, get organic soil. You can get it from an organic farm. You'll need the right compost and other ingredients to make your plantings successful. All the information you need is in gardening books. Your librarian or garden-club enthusiasts know the right titles. Your local Department of Agriculture Extension Division is in your phone book under "United States, Government of." If none of those can be found, write the Department of Agriculture, Washington, D.C.

There are over 120 varieties of tea. You can grow many of them. (Review the food values and minerals in the herbs and botanicals shown in Chapters 4 and 5.) If you work through a club, whoever is in charge will help you identify treasures like comfrey.

Pick it, when you can, with the whole root. Then replant it. If possible, take some of the soil you find around it to replant with it.

You can grow modest amounts of basil, parsley, chive, mint, onion, garlic, shallots and leeks, if you have space. Every one takes only a bit of knowing. For instance, you can buy shallots in the store, as they come, roots and all. Eat the shallots, cutting off and planting the roots with some of the green tubular stem. They'll grow.

Prune shallots in winter. They'll put up new shoots. Eat those and enjoy knowing you are getting wholesome quantities of fresh nutrients, perhaps for the first time. Prune from the outside stems. They're the oldest. Fresh ones keep coming up on the inside and moving out to the edges for you to prune and use.

Don't pull your homegrown parsley out by the root. Snip off the outer growings, as with shallots. The outer sprigs are greenest and richest. If you have space, grow local types of lettuce—Bibb, Boston, whatever. Keep them growing, pruning off the outer leaves for your table. They'll keep replenishing for you.

In general, renew the soil annually. But benefit from reading up on soil maintenance as you expand your new hobby.

Don't try to grow your whole dinner, neither in a window-box nor patio garden. Plan to grow enough for continual addition of a quantity of fresh-grown vitamins and minerals to your table. That's a lot.

Hint: Don't grow beets unless you have lots of space for them. Buy your beets. Look for really *green* beet greens—the greener, the fresher. Use both the greens and beets.

If you have garden space, do grow eggplant and green peppers along with mint, basil and parsley, for beginners. If you have the right conditions—low area and sandy soil—grow celery. Snip off and use the outer celery stalks, letting the plants go on growing. It takes only a few celery plants to supply you all summer long. The dividend is again something fresh-grown for your table.

Don't attempt growing nutritional seeds. Such items as anise seeds, celery seeds and caraway seeds are imported fresh once a year right after harvesting. Keep that in mind as you supply your household needs by shopping Italian, Syrian, Greek or Lebanese specialty groceries. Make friends with the proprietors. They'll keep you alerted to when these items come in fresh. Buy them in quantity when they arrive and store them carefully, well-wrapped, dry and cool until use. You'll know your products are the freshest you can get and you'll also know that they are never more than a year old, which you don't know now.

Don't plant potatoes unless you have lots of space. If you do, here's a hint: Never eat potato sprouts. They are alkaloid and poisonous.

The greens of most other edible tubers are delicious and nutritious, as those of turnips, for instance. In buying turnips, look for *green* greens, not yellowing or pale, which signifies they are stale or pallid in nutrients.

Most health-food stores sell kits for sprouting seeds. Fresh mung, alfalfa, soya and wheat, all of which you can get in a health-food store with instructions for sprouting, provide a great deal of nutrition when sprouted and added fresh to salads, soup, and so on. Sprouting is the easiest way I know to get started growing something fresh for your table, though sprouting all by itself hardly constitutes an exercise regimen.

Let me tell you about a patient I am very proud of. He will read this book with interest, but he is already deeply committed to organically grown food and the rigid avoidance of processed food for health and longevity. He's an inventor, a successful one. Our interest in him centers on his hobby of organic gardening. He practices it on a scale few of us will with the gardens I am urging on you.

Our inventor, sensitive to the fact that nature supplied its own soil builders successfully for centuries before mankind turned to chemicals, nourishes his own large hillside gardens only with natural compost he creates from crop leftovers. These leftovers consist of grass cuttings, fallen leaves, wood chips, vegetable skins, seeds and other residue, even garbage and weeds. He composts these skillfully and feeds these natural nutrients back to his soil in an unending cycle.

My patient has one acre under cultivation, one third devoted to vegetables, another third to fruit trees and the rest to decorative shrubs and a lawn sprinkled with flower beds. The son of homesteaders, he comes by his knowledge of crops and soil naturally. He still uses a hand plough he bought for his first small garden, one that has become over the years an area large enough to supply his own family's needs and those of a selected clientele made up of people who must have organic food for their health.

His quarrel with manmade fertilizers, with their three elements, nitrogen, potassium and phosphate, is that they do not return necessary trace elements to the soil, resulting in nutritionally deficient as well as tasteless fruits and vegetables.

His grandmother lived to be 88, his grandfather 97. His father met death accidentally at 80. My patient expects to break 100. I have examined him and I think he will. His hobby is providing the exercise I am urging, and his garden is providing the nutrients the rest of us would do well to come by if we aspire to reach the century mark.

In her gardens at West Point Farms, Barbara Apisson raises perennially a large assortment of Caucasus favorites, just as Kegan and I did in our smaller garden not far from the New Jersey Palisades. All of us raised—and Barbara still does—staples you'll do well to get to know better.

None of us raised garlic for our own use. It is best imported because that's how to get the best oil values from this valuable planting. Also best purchased as fresh as possible are cloves and German or Mediterranean chamomile, Greek mountain tea, quality vanilla bean, nutmeg, allspice, ginger, coconut, virtually all teas, coffee and cocoa. Chamomile (or camomile) can be grown locally, but I don't recommend the quality of any local product I've been able to find.

Barbara also purchases her supplies of *mahleb* (seeds), *mastica* (mastic leaves), *chaimen* (fenugreek) and the grains she uses. But she does cultivate patches of marigold, petunia, mums, painted daisies, calendula and other flowers to grace the dining tables at West Point Farms. On the food side, she grows chicory from seeds brought from Armenia, rosemary with its hovering sweetness, lavender, thyme, mint, lemon verbena, iris and roses (more decoration). Below, not far from the breeze-catching oak, aged elms, weeping beech, silver and bronze birch, there are ribbons of eggplant, zucchini, Hubbard squash, summer and other squash, cucumber, tomatoes, potatoes, carrots, peas and herbs everywhere.

Barbara raises beans; string beans; corn; many types of lettuce; radishes; parsley; mint; tarragon; basil; sage; strong-scented rue carefully separated from its natural enemy basil; and peppers, bell-shaped, long green, red and others of combined coloration. Peppers are more than abundant at West Point Farms. Careful growing, picking and cool storage give many of Barbara's staples a long season of fresh use, a fundamental of the year-round quality of Barbara's cookery.

Barbara also grows chives; shallots; onions; scallions; local garlic for the West Point Farms dogs and cats; dill; rocca (*arocca, rucala, rauquette*), a kind of cress; *origan* (*Origanum,* a marjoram) and in lower sandier soil celery and celery root. In mid-rows along the slope she has planted melons of many kinds, berries, turnips, parsnip, beet and mustard greens, chard, spinach, cabbages and pumpkin.

With her beloved "family" Elizabeth Kremb at her side,

Barbara carries rainwater to where it is needed or uses long lengths of hose to tap the property wells in dry spells. These tireless women cart humus and ground-up vegetation, weed as needed, work their gardens—great toning for the arms, legs and back and for healthy glowing skin tone.

Their weeding problem is minimized by use of a thin biodegradable material covering the walking areas in low rows. Weeds that would stunt lettuce or cress, stop cucumbers and squash from spreading or take nourishment from zucchini and eggplants, are carefully rooted out and then fed back to the soil as mulch.

Early every spring, radishes, lettuce and herbs begin flowing into the kitchen. By July there are the first tomatoes. Zucchini comes by midseason, eggplant and okra later, then peppers and the first melons. Late summer and early fall bring a wealth of garden yield.

All through late fall and early winter the garden gives fresh bounty to the table. Salads, soups, sauces and entrées are spiked with fresh garden yields. As Barbara does it, the underground plants grow nearly from one end of the year to the next.

Buckets of red apples that have been stored in cold bins all winter long emerge for sauce and for the appetites of the deer who come up to the front lawn to wait for Elizabeth or Barbara, whom they recognize and trust.

Earthworms nourish soil. Chemicals destroy them. Protective plantings, all carefully planned within what appears as a chaotic array of growing produce, keep insects to a minimum, sparing Barbara's naturally grown items for those who dine at West Point Farms. At the same time, sunflowers and other seedbearers are planted to keep the birds coming and happy.

Wood ashes from the fireplace, vegetable leavings, eggshells, coffee grounds, fish bones and other seafood leftovers of the restaurant are saved, permitted to decompose and used as garden feed. By each springtime they restore the soil. Insecticides, pesticides and commercial fertilizers never touch the West Point Farms gardens.

Later, when you read Barbara's recipe for cheese *beurek* and other foods familiar at West Point Farms, know that her chopped parsley, chard, spinach, cress, tomatoes and assorted greens find their way into her soups, salads, entrées and main courses, providing a storehouse of what the body needs for a balanced diet, better health and longer years.

Before we turn to our observations about eating habits in the Caucasus mirrored by Barbara Apisson, let me sum up on exercise: Do and prosper. Amen.

9. Caucasus Diet Fundamentals

Do you remember that splendid Caucasus meal Kegan and I were served by our centenarian hostess, described in Chapter 2? I mention it again because we recently heard of an allegedly "typical" Caucasus fare that does not conform to our experience, our queries, or, for that matter, the experience of the Apissons in their many trips through the area. Nor does it conform to the recollection and practice of numerous Armenians who brought the basic Caucasus diet we know to America and other lands.

Every effort I have made to confirm cornmeal mush as a basic of Caucusus longevity has failed. I cannot understand this conclusion. Corn is plentiful here. It hasn't done much for our statistics. I wish it did contain a magic ingredient to make us live longer if taken daily.

What *might* be recalled usefully in this connection is a time Americans shipped excess corn to India and other areas of famine. The recipient peoples were horrified at the gift. Most of this largesse went unused because, bluntly, use of this grain went against traditions of the "beneficiary" peoples. We do well on nutrient combinations that supply our basic needs within a framework of familiarity. The beauty of the authentic Caucasus diet is that its staples *are* familiar to us and *are* obtainable here.

But we find no heavy use of cornmeal as a feature of the traditional diet. We also dispute the claim that meat is rarely eaten in the Caucasus. Being somewhat scarce, it *is* eaten economically, as we have said, habitually in combination with other foods. If meats are rarely eaten, why does the name for sheep there translate into the words "our roast"?

It is also written that Caucasians eat little fish. The easy availability of a variety of fish in the Black and Caspian seas and the world-renowned Lake Sevan trout belie that. And if coffee is really rare in the area, for what strange purpose does the common phrase *Haigagan Soorj* spring to the lips at mealtimes? That's what they call the Caucasian coffee I drank to my heart's content. Enough on that subject. As I have said earlier, don't be misled.

Sheep's milk yogurt (yes, claims to the contrary notwithstanding, sheep's milk *does* supply much yogurt in the Caucasus), called *madzoon,* is cut with a knife and eaten with a fork as a basic of the Caucasus diet. There is a great variety of vegetables organically grown and eaten. There is a good variety of available greens eaten in salads. These and meats eaten lean and in sensible small quantities (but often enough) are fundamentals. And fruits are grown and eaten fresh or dried, depending on season, as we have told you. Balancing out this excellent nutrient mix is bulgur wheat.

Those are the fundamentals. And just as the actual number of Armenians, or part Armenians, is lost in centuries of intermarriage, of intermingling as invaders swept across this attractive corridor for conquest, so too is the precise history of dietary habits mixed and melded and adapted among the forty or more blended peoples of the Caucasus. But the strong empirical evidence is that survival was taught by the survivors and that the longevity diet is a direct development of the ancient Armenians.

One aspect of Caucasus eating habits we should copy more here, apart from their recipes and nutrient mixes, is concerned with fiber in food.

It was immediately apparent to Kegan and to me that the diet of the long-lived Caucasus peoples is extremely rich in fiber foods. This could have been purely accidental. Or it could have stemmed from wisdom evolved in the centuries-long battle for survival.

Your past familiarity with fiber foods may have been under labels like "bulk" or "roughage." You may not have heard those words for awhile. I believe they went out of vogue because in some people's views some roughage was too rough and some bulk too bulky for digestion and evacuation.

But incoming patients still present me with digestion and evacuation problems to clear up. And I'm here to tell you we saw no roughage or fiber problems in the Caucasus. Lack of roughage in our diet creates mischief within us that is unknown there.

Dr. Jarvis, who popularized Vermont folk medicine, correctly observed that nature opened up the first drugstore. Pioneers saw which plants animals favored for food and medicine. It didn't take people long to copy the animals.

Dr. Jarvis showed independence and wisdom in going his own nutritional way, but I believe his fondness for honey and vinegar as cures for many human ailments took him off the right track. He should have stayed with the plants and vegetables the animals ate for their fiber content and nutrition.

I confess I didn't add all this up in the Caucasus, not even when I saw how fond and devoted people there are of varied fiber foods. I did know those foods were high in nutrient values, and the advantages in picking and eating fresh organically grown foods. And I did see how vigorous physical work helped them burn off their intake without adding weight.

Kegan and I also decided that the nearly universal enthusiasm and good nature of Caucasus people had to do with regularity of bowel habits enjoyed there.

But not until I read Dr. Denis Burkitt's papers on roughage and national eating habits did I find what I regard as a satisfactory explanation for Caucasus health and longevity. Think about this: Dr. Burkitt found that it takes twice as long for food to move through the bowels of Englishmen, eaters of white bread, refined white sugar and other low-bulk foods, as it does to move through the bowels of Africans whose diet is heavy on fiber and whole grains.

To Dr. Burkitt and others turning their attention to this aspect of nutrition, bacterial substances that show up in human waste remain in contact with the lower intestines and colon far longer among Westerners than among Africans, giving us a highly logical explanation for higher rectal–colon cancer rates among Westerners.

Now let's consider the studies of Dr. Ernst L. Wynder of New York's American Health Foundation. He has proved that different bacteria populate the gut of people on a high-fat American diet than, for example, the low-fat, high-vegetable diet of the Japanese. He suggests that the higher amount of cholesterol and bile acids passing through American bowels may account for these bacterial differences.

In the Caucasus, as in Africa and Japan, less animal meats and their fats are consumed than here and in England. Not surprisingly, rectal–colon cancer is nearly unknown in Africa, Japan and the Caucasus.

These studies are more than theory. The fact is, bacteria which thrive on substances derived from human bile and cholesterol have positively been shown to bring about development of a chemical that causes cancer in laboratory animals.

Naturally, this interests me very greatly. You see, I have known for some time the great benefits herbal foods provide through their vitamins and minerals. But I have felt there must be something else in them, something that might be escaping us, that helps restore sick bodies to health. The answer, I am more certain than ever, must lie, too, in the cellulose, pectins, tartrates, citrates and *fiber*—bulk—roughage so abundant in certain vegetables and plants.

Thus Dr. Jarvis would have been more inspired to promote the apple rather than its cider, the edible parts of pollen-laden plants themselves, not the honey. Caucasus food alchemists have habitually strengthened their meals with fiber foods. The result: There is always plenty of roughage pushing the waste through their bowels as with the Africans in Dr. Burkitt's studies. Now there, dear reader, is food for thought!

Related to this subject, dieters, is this information: Studies have shown that a diet heavy in fiber foods pushes significant amounts of ingested calories right through the digestive tract *unabsorbed. When you add enough fiber to your diet, some of the calories you eat really don't count!*

More important, the same fiber foods, when eaten habitually, also appear to supply the motive force to clear foods out of the intestines before excess bile/cholesterol causes the chemical action that spawns cancer-causing agents in the lower bowel. Medical scientists are turning up evidence that fiber-swept bowels are protected not only from rectal–colon cancers but cancers of the pancreas, kidney and elsewhere.

Remarkably, whether they knew what they were doing or not, survival-wise Caucasus aborigines, watching animal habits centuries before Dr. Jarvis's Vermonters did, must have seen how animals favored roughage—fiber—especially to relieve distress. The Caucasians learned their lesson well. Their life-saving lesson, I believe, needs to be relearned in America today.

Fiber does make a difference. Again and again I have seen poor dietary records turned around and health improved significantly when fiber was added to the daily diet in good quantity for a clean sweepdown of the bowels before trouble-making chemicals could form and foul up the body's system of waste disposal.

So if you enjoy bakery products daily, like your steak or lobster, favor processed white flour and white sugar products but hate vegetables, whole-grain foods, fruity pulp, raw or undercooked root foods, legumes, herbs and botanicals, please do some new thinking about it.

Remember the "poor" countries around the world, where starvation reduces lifespan, but where abundant available fiber, consumed to fill hungry guts, prevents diseases among them that find us terribly vulnerable.

Wonder why we're getting fatter as a nation? Wonder why fiber has fallen from favor here? Has faddist reading convinced you that carbohydrates are the villain, not just fat? If so, think about this: In "uncivilized" parts of the world, people eat large quantities of chewy carbohydrates along with those fiber foods they also consume in large quantities. And these people know nearly no obesity, stroke, cancer, heart disease, ulcers, varicose veins, colitis, appendicitis or diverticulitis.

An exaggeration? On May 22, 1971, the *British Medical Journal* took note that a high incidence of these conditions is seen only in *economically developed countries*. Almost a year later, in the April 15, 1972, issue, the journal carried the recommendation of Drs. Burkitt and Painter that diet should be unrefined and should include plenty of vegetation, or roughage.

This is quoted in *The Lancet,* December 22, 1973: "The extreme commonness of obesity of Western countries may be related to the fact that most dietary carbohydrate is refined and fiber-depleted." In this article, by Dr. K. W. Heaton of the Bristol Royal Infirmary, we also read, "I suggest that foods from which fiber has been removed cause overnutrition and that starch and sugar are non-fattening when eaten with their natural component of fiber."

Dr. Heaton's words have been ignored, I suppose, because there is little romance in roughage and no charisma in the whole shoddy subject of proper bowel function.

In still more recent tests, people were fed increasing amounts of fiber as the caloric content of their stool was progressively measured. The results were fascinating. It was found that eating more fiber in fat-rich diets caused more calories, more fat and more cholesterol to be lost by excretion. *Increasing fiber lowered the ability of fattening food to fatten people.* Does this give you a persuasive perspective on the Caucasus habit of eating fiber foods in great amounts in their varied daily salads?

The studies I've mentioned are supported by still others. When subjects who ate whole natural foods including whole-grain breadstuffs were compared with controls who were fed processed foods including refined white bread, it was found that those eating the natural foods excreted an average of 321 more calories a day than the controls.

It was also shown that people eating regular amounts of natural food including fiber averaged 100 calories a day less absorption from the same foods eaten by controls minus the fiber foods. In a year, that alone would make the fiber-food eaters ten pounds lighter than the others.

As best as I can reckon, people on an average American diet probably consume less than one gram a day of fiber. Many get much less because of biases and hates. Caucasus people we studied consume about thirty grams of fiber a day. That's an impressive difference. I see them as better able than we to dispose of calories, cholesterol and total stool output before the chemical changes that generate cancer-causing chemicals in the intestines.

Surely, the fiber facts provide incentive to modify your diet! Even if you can't or won't get *your* fiber consumption up to thirty grams a day, you'll accomplish a great deal if you get it to twenty.

Stop shunning whole, coarse foods. Add all-bran, wheat or rice bran to foods you prepare. Fix breads and cereals at home, using unrefined source materials. Use not just extracts, but the pulp and bulkage of the herbs and botanicals you found in Chapters 4 and 5, and others we'll mention. As we've said, eat the seeds, vegetables, grains and fruits whose pectin, fiber, carbohydrate acids and salts are naturally balanced and vital to your total diet. Do your level best to plan your menus around edible fiber.

We have already touted these same foods for their vitamin and mineral content. Reinforcing that rationale, persuasive enough by itself, is the ability of fiber foods to prevent or at least diminish obesity and disease.

We don't know everything—we're a long way from that. For instance, our knowledge thins when it comes to understanding paciferans, factors of the outer coverings of foods such as grains. They seem to have a lot to do with our personal immune systems, bolstering them, but we haven't figured out how, or how to help them be more effective or how to avoid interfering with their fine work.

No, we don't have all the answers. Those who may choose to attack my reasoning don't either. But a prudent reader, fed up with drugs, fads or simply with how he or she feels on the typical American diet, will surely see merit in giving natural foods a good solid try. Now that you know the Caucasus boasts so many more centenarians than our civilization, doesn't it all make more and more sense?

When I married Kegan Sarkisian, I knew more about how the Eskimo ate than the Armenians. My years of nutrition study and university travels supplied me with some far-out recipes. I knew the food habits of the Orient, had enjoyed Spanish-style cookery in California, the New England cuisine, knew a good deal about Midwest meals and, doing medical time in the South, the secrets of its green vegetables, seafood, chicken and pork. But I vowed that my husband must have his own kind of food and learned there were no books to study. So I collected recipes from his friends and their wives at Armenian picnics, affairs and homes. Gradually, I learned which herbs and which spices distinguished each gourmet treat.

But whatever my informants told me, storekeepers called these items by different names—or, as with pink lentils, they laughed and couldn't remember when they had carried them last. It was a rare specialty or ethnic store that carried what I was looking for, and poor Kegan always had to come along to translate. Luck was spotty. If I found *tahini,* there was no *petmez.* If I located *tarama* after a weary search, *bulgur* was clean off the shelf. *Chaman* (fenugreek) was an impossible dream. Leeks, when found, cost a fortune. Curly dry German parsley was plentiful but the very green broad-leaf Italian type, just right in salads, was hard to come by, as was celery root. A Greek store, found after a long search, had *filo (phyllo),* another sold *kadayif.* But we had to settle for ready-made *baklava, kadayif* (nut-stuffed), *soudjuk* and *lokhoum,* all under their Greek names, at that.

Except in rare Armenian shops, under no name and in no shop did we find *basterma* or *soudjuk,* spiced meats that Kegan spoke of with reverence. Finding an Armenian shop was an event. We left loaded with Kegan's herb finds of sumac (*sumak, sumakh, aghdor, Barberis,* barberry), fresh tarragon, *mahlab (mahleb),* tasty pine nuts and fine-powdered Oriental coffee and chicory.

The first yogurt I purchased may have been old. I couldn't stand the taste. Kegan explained how to make it, but my first tries were disasters. I ruined several successive batches by inoculating the milk when it was still too hot, killing the delicate bacteria. Then I let it cool too much before adding the culture, so the yogurt never developed. Finally, I got the hang of it. Soon Armenian guests were praising its texture, and what I came to appreciate was the acidic quality of my homemade *madzoon.* I earned my spurs when a visiting French scientist pronounced my yogurt the best he had tasted in America.

As I said, there were no books—that is, until 1949, when a group of Armenian women assembled their combined recipes in a spiral-wired booklet called *Treasured Armenian Recipes.* Because Armenian history is so full of venture and go, this collection evokes Damascus, Bagdad, Alexandria and the historic names of Alexander the Great, the Phoenicians, Roman legions and Marco Polo, each charmed by recipes in the collection.

Some of these recipes and more, which Barbara and I will carefully unfold to you, have found their way from the Caucasus to

India, the Middle East and, by many a strange route, to most parts of the world, renamed, shaded, adapted, but with methods and nutrients basically intact.

Recent "secrets" books ascribing the centenarian state of the Caucasus to vegetarianism are as untrue, Armenians agree, as the notion that cornmeal does it!

An absence of junk foods is a key, of course, but the real secret is variety—*all* of nature's best, not just some of it. Meats are used sparingly and fiber foods generously, depositing their vitamin and mineral riches before they provide their second great service of cleaning Caucasians of troublemakers.

History supports the belief that wheat as we know it today started in the Caucasus. It has been cultivated for centuries in Edenland, eaten as *bulgur,* hot sun dried, naturally processed, stored year-round and ground just before using.

Bulgur is fine-ground and kneaded as *kufta* (balls), mixed with chick-peas or meat, and often stuffed. Freshly coarse-ground, the product makes *bulgur* pilaf. *Gorgod* is the large plain whole wheat, a favorite in winter puddings, served November and December right through the holidays.

See also *anoushabour,* a Yule treat in Armenian households the world around, used, too, in Lent, warming the heart and filling the stomach when no meat is eaten by the devout.

Rice pilaf has been a favorite there for centuries. I believe with Kegan that it arrived overland by caravan from the Orient, proving that Caucasus people, themselves an inspiration to the world, knew when to borrow a good thing.

Rice is the chief stuffing for *sarma,* also called grape-vine-leaf *sarma, derevi dolma* or *yalanchi dolma,* eaten with gusto wherever there are Armenians. Oats, barley, millet, buckwheat, rye and a number of kinds of corn are known to grow in the Caucasus. Six-grain breads are a tradition there.

As I have tried to emphasize, meals are mixtures. On my first Caucasus day I had beans, *bulgur,* lamb and vegetables (many kinds), whole-grain breadstuffs, Armenian flatbread, *madzoon* and lots of *kefir* to drink, as it was broiling hot travelling through southern Russia to the first hills of the Caucasus.

The food kept coming in unending variety—melon, grapes, pears, apples, peaches, cherries, plums and apricots, all still fresh in late summer. The last three, like wheat, originated there. It was too late in the year for us to see green nuts growing, but we had those traditional source foods (also quince) in homemade conserves. Pomegranates were still on the trees when the snows came. They were great red balls. Pomegranate is ubiquitous there, eaten fresh and used as juice. Its seeds are crushed into dark sauces served with fish, especially Lake Sevan trout. The seeds, also served in salads and vegetables, provide more roughage loaded with nutrients.

Caucasus citrus, grown near the Black Sea, is scarce in fall and winter. Armenians use pomegranate as a substitute. In late spring and early summer they use the juice of green immature grapes in salads and vegetable dishes for the sourness they like.

They also concoct mature grape concentrate which they use much of the year. Cider and grain vinegars are known, but most of their vinegar comes from wine.

Farmers' markets are everywhere, bursting with produce. When I saw my first cabbage, as large as four human heads, I called Kegan over. The farmers weren't showing off. All their cabbages were that big, some bigger.

Tomato, like its botanical cousin the potato, is heavily grown and eaten there. Tomatoes and their natural fiber greeted us at every lunch and dinner, in salads, served as side dishes, and as substitutes for vegetables or mixed with them in cooking.

Often tomatoes come accompanied by long boats of a cress they call lettuce, or with salad greens, raw and undressed for extra roughage.

You know our habit of snacking up on crackers and salted things with our liquor. Their habit, when drinking, is to snack up on tomatoes. The Caucasus version of the tavern free lunch is all the fiber you can eat, obviously reducing the caloric effect of the drinking. Salted pretzels won't do that for you.

Far from being vegetarians, Caucasus folk insinuate meats and other animal products into everything—broths and stocks are used in pilafs, in cooking vegetables and as an ingredient in sauces and gravies. Meat is mixed with cheeses and is apt to show up from one end of a meal to another, in every course. Meat can turn up in modest quantities in yogurt, *kefir,* dried yogurt farina called *targhana* (used in soups), and in strained cheeses, cream-cheese style, pot, farmer's or cottage.

Then there are the egg dishes. Eggs go into everything, just as meats do. You can't imagine how many vegetable dishes there are in the Caucasus that also contain meat, eggs or meat and eggs.

No edible part of an animal goes unused. Feet, neck and head of the chicken, as well as beef and veal bones, enrich their soups and sauces. Animal organs go into gourmet dishes, sausage and preserved spiced-meat concoctions. Intestines are cleaned and used as sausage casings.

Watermelon is not only familiar as dessert; some of the rind is used as an ingredient in conserves and some as roughage in side dishes.

All kinds of seeds are eaten. Women trying to become pregnant chew seeds long and carefully. Dried and toasted seeds are common in winter. Sunflower seeds abound as a source rich in unsaturated oil. Squash, sesame, poppy, caraway, anise, celery and herbal seeds like coriander are popular natural food additives.

We saw squash roasted, steamed and even skewered in shish kabob. We saw squash served in soups, as a vegetable with meats, in Lenten dishes, in conserves and preserved for winter. Nothing is wasted. Starvation and survival under siege taught early Caucasians respect for all nutrients. This respect has given them super-durable bodies.

All kinds of natural aids build up their soils. They use wood ashes for potash and also add humus-composts and animal dung, well-ripened from the year before. They use sand, sea plants, sea-water, fish leftovers, fish from the Black Sea and algae from their ponds. They use lava powders and leftover scraps of *tufa* (a solid mineral the consistency of a moist soft clay underground which they cut to size, allow to harden and use much the way we use cinder block).

The only protective sprays they use are made from the same flowers that protect their plantings from insects.

That's as far as I'll go in describing Caucasus health habits. Obviously, many are easy to incorporate. Some are not. All those you can make a part of your day-to-day routine are worth trying. Learn *something* from this survival regimen you have been reading about, the more the better, even if you can't use it all. Here are my summarized recommendations, representing what I believe you *can* use from what we have been describing.

Caucasus Diet Habits To Copy

1. Dine graciously. Enjoy mealtimes. Dress up to eat now and then. Make meals special. When relaxation is a necessity, on the other hand, don't be rigid about dress. Avoid quick eating. Don't eat on your feet or on the run. Use mealtimes to break a day's pace, not as part of the rush.

2. Eat something fresh at every meal, fresh fruit with breakfast, salad with lunch and dinner. Eat lots of greens. When deciding what to prepare or to order, skip anything but the greens.

3. Vary meals by varying recipes. Don't get locked into a few favorite staples. Experiment. Create surprises. Even small

changes make a big difference. Consciously construct in every menu an assortment which, in total, adds up to a fully balanced diet, generous in the varied nutrients needed to sustain and advance body health. If you're not doing this now, you're simply not providing the nutrient balance your family needs. An approach that adds sensible snacks to smaller balanced meals is well worth the effort.

Remember that grain foods are interchangeable with the bean group; pilafs can alternate with potatoes and stuffings; breadstuffs are the first items to eliminate in a quest for variation. Omitting bread items, fill in with mixtures: vegetable/grain/pilaf/meat or fish concoctions. Your imagination in mixing, Caucasus-style, is the key to innovative menus.

4. Fit into your daily plan calcium-rich dairy foods. Take some yogurt before bedtime. Also work it into your cookery, soups and snacks. Get into the between-meal snack habit of cheeses, not pastries; raw fruits and vegetables, not candies; natural foods, not prepared processed items. To get the calcium your body needs, take our suggestions on *tan*, *kefir*, whole milk and buttermilk to heart. Another way: Add dabs of cottage or farmer's cheese to your salads. Recheck Chapters 4 and 5 for your calcium and chromium sources. Emphasize those foods in your menus.

5. Another must for every day is vegetables, preferably fresh. Whoever set the rule of one vegetable and a potato per main course put us on the wrong track. Certainly it's more trouble, but two, three or more vegetables served in small quantities each, in addition, if you like, to a small, lightly steamed potato, provide a far wider spread of food values than just one vegetable served with a potato. Remember, use little or no water with vegetables. Try sautéing lightly. Eat as many as you can raw.

6. Use nature's supplements as well as the supplementation I have suggested in my Chapter 5 vitamin/mineral chart. Eat food yeasts, *petmez*, sunflower and other seeds, nuts and all the source foods we mentioned earlier, including pollen. Health-food stores sell pollen granules. It is also available in unrefined honey. But in the Caucasus and at West Point Farms, Armenians pick pollen-laden flowers fresh in the fields and gardens. Barbara Apisson steeps fresh whole flowers, many kinds, in water, bringing the brew to a boil, lets it stand and "absorb," and drinks it. The whole family does. Fresh floral teas are something to learn about. They provide fresh pollen, the way the bees get it. Surely, you can do that, too. Just so, you can eliminate junk foods as we've urged, thereby providing the budgetary support for purchases of the right foods your body needs.

7. Read and use our Chapter 10 menus for taking off weight.

Read and *enjoy* using Barbara Apisson's Chapter 11 maintenance menus, an open sesame to nutritious dining that gives you pleasure as well as health.

If you have decided you are worth the trouble of giving our regimen a try, the seven steps outlined above are the way to get organized and get started. For overweight readers, the starting line is the next chapter.

10.

Our Weight-Off Diet

We are about to serve up two weeks of weight-off meals. Before we do, let me say again to would-be dieters that if you are going to try ours, *especially* if you have dieted before, please see your doctor first. A previous diet, especially one of those I complained about earlier in the book, may have gotten you into trouble or set you up for it. Faulty diets can aggravate the kidneys, heart and liver, bring on anemia, or leave you with fragile bones and/or emotional problems.

So before embarking even on our diet, which I expect to reduce obesity without attacking your health, get examined first. Be sure your present health permits you to diet. If your health is not up to par, follow orders and get well before starting our regimen.

When you do begin, support your diet with the modest vitamin and mineral supplementation recommended in our Chapter 5 chart! *And* get into exercise on an ascending scale to tone up your body and support the development of the new you. You'll find in our diet an ample amount of valuable fiber foods that will discourage constipation and its hazards to successful healthy dieting. In short, you are not simply to follow our menus, you are to follow our entire recommended course of action which, taken as a whole, can put you on the right track to longer life, improved health and the side reward of improved sexual performance.

Caucasus peoples are blessed with a complete natural diet. Of course, they are not trying to lose weight on that regimen. So, of necessity, our weight-off version of the Caucasus diet, which you are about to read, obviously doesn't include everything you'll find in our Chapter 11 maintenance meals. You'll make up the important differences with vitamin and mineral supplementation.

All right, you have been examined. Your doctor pronounces you sound. With or without reservations, he tells you to try our diet if you like. Here's how we want you to do it. After two weeks of our diet menus without cheating, you will have taken off at least ten pounds. At that point, we would like to see you switch over to Chapter 11 maintenance meals for two or three weeks, continuing your exercise on a rising curve of activity. Then, if you would like to shed another ten pounds, go back to our Chapter 10 weight-off regimen for another two weeks. By moving back and forth between the weight-off menus and maintenance meals, you can (1) set your own personal timetable for the amount of weight you want to remove and the length of time you want it to take, and (2) between weight-off periods nutritiously maintain your losses while (3) you acquire expertise in Caucasus-style cookery, your open sesame to a longer, healthier existence.

Switching back and forth between our diet and maintenance meals will, if you are serious about this, not rapidly but eventually bring you to your ideal weight, which we define as the lowest weight you want and can maintain.

By the time you are approaching that point, the Caucasus habits we're urging on you should have taken hold. Moderate to careful practice of these new nutrition habits, with as few as possible lapses into processed food, refined white-sugar and white-flour products, will add both years and enjoyment of them.

Get a kitchen scale if you don't have one now. It should measure weight in grams. But for readers with scales in ounces, we're giving our weights in both. Incidentally, when we propose tbsp. (tablespoon) or tsp. (teaspoon), we have in mind for you to use a level one, not a heaping one. If you don't already own them, buy measuring spoons of the different sizes you'll need, all joined together in a nest for convenience. Any hardware or kitchen-utensil store has the set.

Before we get into the menus, a little straight talk, if you please. The look these days is trim, right? But if you had been prepared to give your all to be thin, you would *be* thin. Right? The point is, no pep talk from me at this point can change that unless the first nine chapters of this book have impressed you that *this is the way*.

People are scarcely alike in their attitudes, problems, paces, styles, ambitions, hangups, indulgences, needs for reward, needs to punish themselves and others, and in the ways in which they use or refuse food from infancy on, for compensation, for power, for all manner of purposes and cross-purposes.

Whatever your character makeup and body state, unless you

share the same physical problem that keeps me at top weight in my acceptable range (and it's a struggle at that), you can take off weight—if you will!

I have had patients in thirty seconds turn on the enthusiasm to set out along the road to accomplish it, and then follow through to success. I have seen others take a lot longer but get there. Still others have yet to find within themselves the motivation to remake their bodies. That won't surprise people who have dieted before, lost weight and then gained it back with interest. They know dieting is hard work, fraught with temptation.

But I promise you this: Barbara and I have struggled for many months to create our calorie combinations. We have fought to pare down calories without giving you a regimen that will either defeat or coddle you. We have made and corrected mistakes and lost sleep worrying through the right combinations with nutritional staying power yet which were low enough in calories and carbohydrates to work for you to the end.

We have been rewarded and even surprised at how well Caucasus food and methods have adapted to the demands we placed on them. I promise ten pounds off, but I hope for more. And I'm happy to assure you that you won't starve. These meals provide a lot to eat.

Having said a pep talk won't help, I can't resist these next few words. I believe in the power of meditation, reflection and self-analysis. The following four steps in that direction may help start you down the road to self-improvement:

1. *Determined Self-Awareness.* Vague wishing doesn't get you far, but deepening attention to the YOU in you, purposeful thinking over what you are all about, what's right about and for you, what's wrong about and for you, will accomplish much and provide the inducement for you to make a dietary investment in a better you.

2. *Self-Communication* is the technique for achieving self-awareness. Speak out orally—declare yourself *to* yourself. Also, write down your thoughts for later consultation. Put what you are, what you want, what you need into real spoken and written words. Tell yourself what needs to be changed to make you happy. Make a commitment to yourself to work to make it happen. Write a program.

3. *Self-Renunciation* starts you toward a new you. Be prepared to give up something to gain something better. Spell it out again and again. What will you give for a beautiful body? Junk food? Effort? Determination?

4. *Imitation.* Think thin. Select a slender person you ad-

mire and decide to be like that person. Imitate whatever and whomever you most admire for the qualities (and quantities) you find most appealing.

Before you decide I've become unhinged, there's a practical side to meditating. Studies show people can lose up to one hundred calories from one hour of good solid meditation. How's that for a bonus for a dieter? It may help to try this yourself:

1. Self-Awareness
2. Self-Communication
3. Self-Renunciation
4. Imitation

Don't think it can't be done. It's done all the time. Queen Esther did it for six months—rubbed down, shaped up, dieted, mobilized her deepmost resources and won a king. You can do as much by taking full charge of yourself and *starting* now.

Now let's get ready to look at our weight-off days. You should be able to prepare everything in these diet meals from the included instructions. There's meat—but not excessive meat. You'll get the rest of your needed protein by the classic Caucasus method of mixing proteins. Calories per day vary from some 500 on the low side to about 900 on the high side. Carbohydrates vary from 40 to 60 grams a day.

A word about shopping. We've already suggested buying fresh, buying only what you need, using it up and buying again. Stick to that formula in your diet purchases as a safeguard against loss of food values. These diet meals will require forethought in shopping your needs. Plan your acquisitions in writing. Check them off as you get them. Walking from store to store to find them all fits our exercise regimen.

Particularly if you work during the day, your shopping trips will have to cover your needs for all three meals. Also, you must arrange to carry and store ingredients for some unusual lunches or else be able to get back to home base for lunch. It's not likely you can buy many of these lunches out, although you might, with persistence, buy parts of them and carry the rest.

Fitting these or any dieting requirements into social and economic needs takes determination and intelligence. It can mean staying up late to prepare the night before and refrigerate. I wish it were easy. If it were, we would all be sylphs. But remember—you're in charge and you're worth it.

One more point: In my calorie counts, I have taken into

account sticky foods that cling to pots, as well as calories that go up in smoke or evaporate in cookery or preparation. Our calorie count is based on what gets into you.

You have seen how important fish and seafood are as low-calorie protein. Because they are such important sources, Barbara and I have compiled the following shopping list of low-calorie fish, seafood and garnishes for both. These are items you can combine any way you like to add up to the right number of calories and carbohydrates called for in two places in the diet, providing both low-calorie nutrition and acceptable flavoring.

Omitted from the shopping list are halibut, herring, mackerel, pollock, sablefish, salmon (all but pink or humpback), sardines (all but Norwegian in tomato sauce), trout (except brook), shad, swordfish, weakfish and whitefish. They're all too high in calories for our list. I've left oysters out, too; they're too high in carbohydrates (CHO). The figures for selected fish and seafood are based on four-ounce portions of raw meat only unless otherwise stated.

As I indicated, there are two places in the diet meals that refer you to the shopping list for your choice of selections to make up 175 or 180 calories and 2 to 3 grams CHO. But that's not the only reason I have compiled this list. I wanted you to have a place to turn to for substitution where necessary if you can't find items called for, with the simple arithmetic provided to guide you to intelligent choices. But there's another reason. Between official dieting sessions, it's good to know this basic group of nutritious low-calorie, low- (or no) carbohydrate foods. This is an excellent group to get to know well, not necessarily as part of a strict structured diet, but simply when you ought to prune calories because you've overdone it at the table.

A word of caution: I must strongly urge that you *not* use this shopping list to excess. Use it only when directed to it in the diet or in what we hope will be infrequent shopping emergencies during the diet period. Do *not* make up your own total diet from it. Used that way, it would be faddish and dangerous.

Shopping List—Fish, Seafood and Extras

4 oz.	CAL	CHO	4 oz.	CAL	CHO
CARP	126	0	HADDOCK	90	0
CLAM	93	1.5	HAKE	84	0
COD	89	0	LOBSTER	108	.4
CRAB, steamed	106	.6	PERCH, OCEAN	108	0
CRAPPIE	90	0	PERCH, WHITE	134	0
CRAYFISH	82	1.4	PERCH, YELLOW	103	0
FLOUNDER, filet	90	0	PICKEREL	95	0

PIKE, BLUE	102	0
PORGY	127	0
ROCKFISH	121	2.2
ROE, cod, shad only, baked or broiled	143	2.2
SALMON, pink or humpback only	135	0
SARDINE, Norwegian in tomato sauce only	124	1.7
SCALLOPS, cooked or steamed	127	0
SEA BASS	109	0
SHRIMP	103	1.7
SMELT	111	0
SNAPPER, red or grey	105	0
SOLE	90	0
SQUID	95	1.7
STURGEON	107	0
TERRAPIN	126	0
TUNA, canned in water	144	0
TROUT, brook only	115	0
TURTLE	101	0

For flavoring any of the above, add the following:
(1 oz. = 28.35 grams; T = Trace)

	CAL	CHO
½ tsp. fresh lemon juice	.66	.2
Tabasco sauce, ¼ tsp.	.75	0
Worcestershire, Heinz, tsp.	2	.5
Parkelp, sprinkle	T	T
if 1 tbsp. veg. oil used to sauté, assume 1 tsp. absorbed	45	0
chili sauce, 1½ tsp.	9	2
1 oz. horseradish	11	2.7
1 large green olive	8	.1
cucumber (⅓ of 7 to 8″ piece)	14	3
1 tbsp. chopped parsley	1	T
1 8″ stalk celery	5	1.6
½ cup lettuce leaves	4	.95
1 cup watercress	6	1
1 cup endive (2.5 oz.)	14	2.9
3 spears asparagus	10	2
½ cup soybean sprouts	19	2
½ cup chard, cooked leaves & stalks	14	2.25

Thus, 4 oz. of tuna meat (144 calories) on ½ cup of lettuce leaves (4 calories, .95 CHO), garnished with 1 tbsp. chopped parsley (1 calorie, T CHO), ½ tsp. fresh lemon juice (.66 calorie, .2 CHO), accompanied by one 8″ celery stalk (5 calories, 1.6 CHO) totals 155 calories and 2.75 CHO. Add .4 oz. of tuna, for instance, to total 175 calories and about 3 CHO if that is your allowance in the diet menu—or if you're substituting for that much.

Day 1 Total Calories: 842 Carbohydrates: 59-60 g.

BREAKFAST	***Serving***	***Calories***	***CHO***
Cantaloupe, thinly sliced	¼ melon	30	7
*_Basterma_ sausage slices OR Canadian bacon	3 thin or 2 medium slices	110	0

**See Chapter 11 recipe*

	Serving	*Calories*	*CHO*
Homebaked low-calorie bread, thinly sliced, OR glutagen-gluten (e.g., Thomas's)	1 slice	40 (35)	7 (5.6)
Herb tea: thyme, Greek mountain or your choice, no sweetener	1 cup	0	0
		180	14 max.

LUNCH

Fresh greens juice with a sprinkle of Parkelp (nutritious flavoring, salt substitute sold in health-food stores). (Blenderize 2 large lettuce leaves, 1 oz. or 29 g. fennel leaves, 1 oz. watercress, 2 oz. or 58 g. parsley with sprig or two of mint. Consume with pulp.) Water to thin. Add cracked ice	in a cup	37	7
Sip above with portion pot cheese	3 tbsp.	33	.5
Select from Shopping List	your choice	175	2-3
Steamed fennel wedges, lower third of vegetable, using upper part in greens-juice blend above	3 tbsp.	14	2
Yogurt (plain only and always)	½ cup	76	6
Herb tea or demitasse	1 cup	0	0
		335	17.5 to 18.5

DINNER

*Roast lamb, no gravy or sauce (your portion), raw weight 2½ oz. or 71 g.	1 slice	130	0
**Bulgur*, simmered in *fat-free chicken stock	3 tbsp.	42	9

**See Chapter 11 recipes*

	Serving	Calories	CHO
Swiss chard, steamed	½ cup	17	3 max.
Fresh or dried apricot compote. Cook lightly in low water or soak overnight without cooking. No sugar	8 halves (medium-sized)	70	16
Herb tea	1 cup	0	0
		259	28 max.

MID-EVENING SNACK

Paupiette d'Agneau (Leftover roast: 1-oz. or 29-g. slice rolled with a lettuce leaf)	1 slice	68	0
Herb tea fizz (choice of herbs) (Fill glass with chipped ice or cubes, adding hot herb tea and seltzer to taste)	1 glass	0	0

Notes: Measure amounts carefully to get proper calorie counts. Gram–ounce equivalents are slightly rounded but close enough to provide correct totals if observed. Make greens juices a must in dieting and in everyday life. It's a lifelong answer to the problem of leaving your needed greens in the salad plate uneaten and it gives you your needed fiber in easy-to-take form. Parkelp, sold at health-food stores, is a nutritious salt substitute and flavoring. We call for it often.

Day 2 Total Calories: 641 Carbohydrates: 74 g.

BREAKFAST	*Serving*	*Calories*	*CHO*
Whole oats, slow cooked in *fat-free chicken stock, using 1.1 oz. or 31 g.		100	17
oats. Grate 1 whole small apple on		35	8
top and add 4 tbsp. half'n'half cream	¾ cup	80	4
	(cooked)	215	29

**See Chapter 11 recipe*

LUNCH	*Serving*	*Calories*	*CHO*
Tomato-*tarama* cocktail (½ cup tomato juice, 1 tbsp. well-mashed pink roe and chipped ice blended or well shaken in a cocktail shaker)	6-oz. glass	35	4.5
Braised tongue (¾ oz. or 21 g.)	1 slice	51	0.08
Stuffed tomato salad (Quarter without cutting through a small raw tomato. Top with ¼ cup chopped celery, chopped cabbage or chopped cauliflower, or combine for same total amount. Add 2 slivered radishes, ½ tsp. sunflower oil, a squeeze of lemon. Serve on bed of finely chopped dill and lettuce greens)	as described	85	12.5
Herb tea fizz in glass or demitasse		0	0
		171	17

DINNER			
Tossed green salad (Chopped dill, lettuce and mint greens tossed with chopped onion, scallion or chives to taste, total ½ cup. Add ½ tsp. unsaturated oil, squeeze of lemon, vinegar or *Verjuice. Toss all well)		35	2
Roast turkey breast, no gravy, no sauce, 1.4 oz. or 40 g., raw weight	1 slice	70	0
Baked potato, medium to small, 3 to 4 drops of Tabasco, a sprinkle of Parkelp	1 potato	60	11
Steamed fresh asparagus	10 thin spears	35	5 max.
Herb tea or demitasse		0	0
		200	18 max.

**A commercial product, flavoring of nutritional value*

MID-EVENING	*Serving*	*Calories*	*CHO*
Yogurt-fresh strawberry fizz (Mix 3 tbsp. yogurt, ½ cup ripe strawberries, mashed or blenderized. Add seltzer and pour over chipped ice)		55	9

Day 3 Total Calories: 717 Carbohydrates: 63 g.

BREAKFAST	*Serving*	*Calories*	*CHO*
Blueberries or wild berries	½ cup	42	10 max.
1 large boiled egg, a sprinkle of Parkelp	1	70	0
Dry lightly toasted low-calorie bread (As in Day 1 menu)	1 slice	40	7 max.
Tea, herb tea or black coffee	1 cup	0	0
		152	17 max.

LUNCH			
Greens and tomato juice cocktail (Blenderized selected greens as in Day 1 menu, add ¼ cup tomato juice, serve on chipped ice)	6-oz. glass	50	10
Select from Shopping List	your choice	180	3 max.
Herb tea or demitasse		0	0
		230	13

DINNER

Poached Cod, Mandarin Supreme (3 oz. or 90 g. filet of cod, raw weight; 1 tangerine peeled, fingered and laid across fish. Top with 2 tbsp. tangerine or lime juice; ½ tsp.

	Serving	*Calories*	*CHO*
chopped parsley. Poach in ¼ to ½ cup fat-free chicken stock, add Par-kelp to taste. Poach to taste)	1 serving	140	10
Hot cooked cucumber-endive-green pepper salad. (Add to sliced vegetables 1 tsp. finely chopped scallions, a few drops of vinegar. Cook all lightly in fat-free chicken stock, topped for serving with few drops of unsaturated vegetable oil)	2 tbsp.	55	3
Clove Cinnamon Peach Compote (poach one 4-oz. or 115-g. peach, 2″ in diameter in enough chicken stock to cover; sprinkle lightly with powdered cinnamon, adding a few whole cloves)		35	8
Herb tea or demitasse		0	0
		230	21

MID-EVENING

Pink *kefir* or buttermilk (Mix 1 tsp. beet juice with 1 cup *kefir* or buttermilk. Add seltzer, ice chips or cubes)	tall glass	105	12 max.

Day 4 Total Calories: 789 Carbohydrates: 40 g.

BREAKFAST	*Serving*	*Calories*	*CHO*
Baked puffed fruit omelet (Beat 1 medium egg yolk, fold in 2 tbsp. cottage cheese, 1 small grated ripe apple, 1 tbsp. whipped butter, and finally beaten egg white. Bake until firm and brown-topped)		212	9

	Serving	*Calories*	*CHO*
Cider fizz (Pour ½ cup natural apple cider over chipped ice, add seltzer)	1 glass	60	14
Herb tea or black coffee	1 cup	0	0
		272	23

LUNCH

Caucasus borscht soup (Mix 1 cup fat-free chicken stock; ¼ cup fresh grated beets; ¼ tsp. fresh lemon juice; a sprinkle of Parkelp. Poach 15 minutes. Chill. Rub bowl with fresh garlic. Garnish with thin cucumber slice, add a sprinkle of chopped dill and mint. Top with 1 tsp. yogurt when serving.	1 bowl	12	1.5
Mixed green salad (Combine cress, lettuce, radish, sliced or chopped; a few cooled, cooked string beans; ½ tsp. chopped chives, onion or scallions; a few sprinkles of dill or your favorite herb(s); a squeeze of lemon juice or a few drops of vinegar; a sprinkle of Parkelp to taste)	equivalent of 1 cup	15	T
Kufteh with mushrooms, Burgundy wine (Serving consists of four 1-oz. or 30-g. balls composed of 2 parts lean-ground veal or beef, 1 part ground lamb, 1 part fine-ground liver, well-mixed. Poach *kufteh* in fat-free chicken stock, adding 2 tsp. Burgundy wine to stock. Simmer 15 minutes after adding 3 sliced mush-			

**See Chapter 11 recipe, too*

	Serving	*Calories*	*CHO*
rooms. Diet serving: 3 mushrooms, 4 balls, ¼ cup broth. NOTE: For a light, tender *kufteh* ball, add 1 tsp. fine-grated onion when mixing)		160	T
Herb tea or demitasse		0	0
		187	2 max.

DINNER

	Serving	*Calories*	*CHO*
Paupiette-Filet Sole Dolma (Marinate 1 large cucumber in white wine and chopped onions for 1 to 2 hours. Parboil cucumber until soft. Roll sole filet, raw weight 135 g. or 4.7 oz., around butcher stick. Stuff stick with fish into hollow tube of cucumber. Poach 5 minutes or more, to taste)		125	5 max.
Caucasus caviar as garnish for *dolma* (Pound 1 tbsp. *tarama* with 1 tbsp. bread crumbs. Diet serving is 1 tsp. only)		16	2
Tossed green salad (Combine alfalfa sprouts, chopped lettuce and dill, a sprinkle of Par-kelp, vinegar, a few drops salad oil. Chill on chilled salad plate)		25	T
Steamed spinach, chard or lettuce	½ cup	20 max.	3 max.
Minted greens cocktail (Blenderize ¼ raw zucchini with 2 slices cucumber, ½ green pepper. Add chipped ice, seltzer, sprig of mint. Use fresh mint when available, otherwise dried)	1 glass	16	3
Herb tea or demitasse		0	0
		207	13

MID-EVENING SNACK	*Serving*	*Calories*	*CHO*
Health nut cup (Combine 1 tbsp. fresh pumpkin/squash seed kernels; 1 tbsp. fresh sunflower seed kernels; 8 shelled pistachio nuts; a pinch of Par-kelp; a pinch of alfalfa sprouts)		75	2
Natural cheddar (.4 oz. or 11.4 g.)	1 slice	48	0
		123	2

Day 5 Total Calories 770–785 Carbohydrates 63–69.5 g.

BREAKFAST	*Serving*	*Calories*	*CHO*
Fresh fruit (1 small apple OR 1 medium-size ripe peach OR 1 medium tangerine OR ¼ cup melon balls (51 g. or 1.75 oz.) (Slice, chill and serve)		35	8
Low-calorie bread (see Day 1 menu)	1 slice	40 max.	7 max.
Tan, a dairy drink (½ cup yogurt blended with water and ice OR *kefir* OR buttermilk OR ½ cup chilled goat or soya milk)	1 glass 1 cup 1 serving	75 (90) (80)	6 (12) (5.5)
Your choice of unsweetened beverage		0	0
		150-165	20.5-27

LUNCH			
½ medium grapefruit		35-40	10 max.
Fresh steamed or poached scallops (45 g. or 1.6 oz. raw weight)	1 cup	112	0
Baked potato, medium-small	1	60	10
Tossed green salad (Combine greens, cucumber, a few			

	Serving	*Calories*	*CHO*
drops fresh salad oil, lemon or vinegar, dill, a sprinkle of Parkelp)	1 plus cup	35	2
Noncaloric beverage of choice	1 cup	0	0
		247 max.	23

DINNER

Tomato juice, a lemon wedge, a sprinkle of Parkelp. (Suggestion: Take with 2 fish-liver-oil capsules)	½ cup	24	4.5
½ broiled chicken (207 g. or 7.3 oz., raw), rubbed with garlic, basted with chicken stock	as described	280	0
Hearts of artichoke, steamed or poached in fat-free chicken stock	2 hearts	14	5
Brussels sprouts, steamed or poached in chicken stock	7 to 8, small	55	10
Noncaloric beverage of choice (Drink coffee or demitasse sparingly. Lean more toward herbal teas)	1 cup	0	0
		373	19.5

MID-EVENING

Herb tea fizz		0	0

Day 6 Total Calories: 754 Carbohydrates: 44 g.

BREAKFAST	*Serving*	*Calories*	*CHO*
Fresh fruit (¼ cup fresh strawberries, slightly crushed (37 g. or 1.3 oz.) OR slices of ¾ of 1 ripe peach)	as described	27	3
1 tbsp. yogurt topping	1 tbsp.	9	0.7

	Serving	*Calories*	*CHO*
Garnish with a sprinkle of nutmeg, cinnamon or clove plus 1 tbsp. fresh sesame seeds	1 tbsp.	22	0.8
Scramble 1 small egg beaten with ½ tbsp. of half'n' half cream, a pinch of Parkelp and a pinch of chopped parsley and tarragon. Cook in double boiler, stir constantly 4 to 6 minutes to desired thickness		76 plus	0.5
Low-calorie bread (see Day 1 menu). May be lightly toasted (prefer warmed, foil-wrapped)	1 slice	40 max.	7 max.
Hibiscus flower blended herb tea, hot. (Blend of hibiscus, clove, rose hip, orange—or available variation)	1 cup	0	0
		174	12

LUNCH

Your choice of soup base, bought in health-food store (a powder with dried nutritive bits and morsels in it). Label shows it free of salt, sugar, preservatives. Add 1 tsp. to 1 cup chicken stock or boiling water and allow to simmer several minutes. (Varieties available: vegetable, onion, celery, protein, beef, chicken, carrot, bean, pea)	1 cup	25	5 max.
Protein salad (Use ¾ cup of leftover turkey or chicken chunked, or chopped liver, seafood or cooked fish. Swirl with a pinch of Parkelp, alfalfa sprouts (just a few), a squeeze of lemon, a few drops of salad oil, pinches of finely chopped scallion, dill, chive, diced celery and chopped lettuce, whichever are available)		150	T

	Serving	*Calories*	*CHO*
Low-calorie fruit loaf (Mix 1 small grated apple or the equivalent in bits of other fruit (pear, citron bits, for instance) with a cup of any whole grain cooked in water; bake until brown and firm in a small baking dish or tin. Add no sugar. Portion is 16 g. or a generous ½ oz.)	1 slice	60	9 plus
Herb tea or demitasse		0	0
		235	14

DINNER

Baked shepherd's pie casserole (To 2 oz. or 57 g. of ground beef add one 4-oz. or 114-g. finely sliced kidney of lamb, ½ tsp. chopped onion and sprinkle on your choice of herbs. Sauté in a few drops of vegetable oil and slowly add ½ cup of fat-free chicken stock. Top with a thin crust of riced potato, using small potato. Brush with a trace of cream or butter to hold moisture. Bake golden-brown)		290	13
Steamed endive, chicory or escarole	1 cup	25	T
Kefir rose (tomato-buttermilk) (½ cup tomato juice, 1 tbsp. *kefir* or buttermilk, sprinkles of alfalfa sprouts, chervil, Parkelp as garnish)	1 glass	30	5

MID-EVENING

Herb tea or demitasse	1 cup	0	0
		345	18

Day 7 Total Calories: 672 Carbohydrates: 69.5 g.

BREAKFAST	*Serving*	*Calories*	*CHO*
Fresh berry broil (¼ cup ripe strawberry halves, topped with ½ tsp. anise seeds, a sprinkle of cinnamon. Broil 1 to 2 minutes and serve hot. Can substitute halved gooseberries if preferred)		14 max.	3
Bacon'n'eggplant (Poach 1 thick slice eggplant in fat-free chicken stock. Serve with 1 slice Canadian bacon or 2 to 3 thin slices Soudjuk—Armenian spiced beef sausage—on platter rimmed with 6 sprigs of fresh garden cress)		77	4
Low-calorie bread (see Day 1 menu)	1 slice	40 max.	7 max.
Herb tea or black coffee		0	0
		131	14

LUNCH	*Serving*	*Calories*	*CHO*
Baked mushroom pie (It's easier to prepare multiple servings but tiny pie plates are available. To ½ cup mushrooms, add ½ tbsp. or 1½ tsp. finely ground millet or **targhana* and 1 cup fat-free chicken stock. Sprinkle on chopped dill, Parkelp. For crust, rice ½ small boiled potato, spread, oven bake and serve)		81	15
Zucchini cheese broil (Poach 168 g. or 5.8 oz. squash slices until slightly *al dente*. Can be done in A.M. or night before. Top with thin			

**Barbara Apisson prepares* targhana *(dried yogurt curd mixed with millet or soy meal or farina) by hand-crumbling when almost sun-dried, for use in soups or as a nutritious snack.*

	Serving	*Calories*	*CHO*
slice of cheddar or brick cheese and broil about 1 minute, or until cheese melts into squash. May be eaten hot or cold.		95	6.5
Herb tea or demitasse		0	0
		176	21.5

DINNER

Roast turkey breast (Approximately 80 g. or 2.8 oz.)	2 slices	140	0
Brown or wild rice pilaf (½ cup rice cooked in fat-free chicken stock, seasoned with Par-kelp to taste)	3 tbsp.	89	18
Steamed or poached broccoli (180 g. or 6.35 oz.)	1 large spear	45	7
(Put 4 g. or .14 oz. whipped butter on broccoli, pilaf, turkey, as desired)	2 pats total	50	T
Diced fresh watermelon (158 g. or 5.3 oz.)	1 cup	41	9
Herb tea fizz or demitasse	1 glass or cup	0	0

MID-EVENING

Seltzer on ice	1 glass	0	0
		365	34

Day 8 Total Calories: 664 Carbohydrates: 25.4–29.4 g.

BREAKFAST	*Serving*	*Calories*	*CHO*
1 large poached or boiled egg	1 egg	75	0
Low-calorie bread or toast (see Day 1 menu)	1 slice	40 max.	7 max.

	Serving	Calories	CHO
Sesame (*tahini*) paste (zero cholesterol) on the bread OR 1 generous tbsp. of sesame seeds	½ tbsp.	25	0.5 max.
Herb tea or black coffee	1 cup	0	0
		140	7.5

LUNCH

	Serving	Calories	CHO
Veal heart or lamb kidney and peppers (Braise an 85-g. or 3-oz. lean kidney or heart in a mix with 1 tbsp. salad oil, ½ cup sliced mushrooms and 1 medium-sized green pepper with center and seeds removed, sliced into small slivers. Season with ¼ tsp. of oregano, ½ tsp. fresh lemon juice, a pinch of Parkelp. Braise; do not overcook)		295	4 max.
Salad (½ thinly sliced cucumber on lettuce with a few drops of vegetable oil and natural cider vinegar)		15	5
Herb tea or demitasse		0	0
		310	9

DINNER

	Serving	Calories	CHO
Poached rock, king or blue crab (85 g. or 3 oz.) OR 1 homemade fish cake, your recipe, same weight, OR equivalent short portion from Shopping List	½ cup	79 (76)	0.4 (4)
Tossed green salad (as in Day 5 menu) OR lettuce greens, cucumber sliced thin, scallion	1 cup	35	2
Lightly poached fennel	½ cup	14	1 max.
Your choice of a noncaloric beverage		0	0
		128	3.4-7.4

MID-EVENING	*Serving*	*Calories*	*CHO*
Cottage cheese and fruit (Mix ½ cup cottage cheese with ½ medium sliced peach or top with ½ small apple, grated)		86	5.5

Day 9 Total Calories: 857 Carbohydrates: 30 g.

BREAKFAST	*Serving*	*Calories*	*CHO*
Viande sautée Armenienne (Mix 37-g. or 1-oz. chopped or diced lamb liver with 155 g. or 5.4 oz. of beef or veal kidney and 29 g. or 1 oz. of lean chopped shoulder lamb or veal. Broil in pan brushed with oil or butter, lightly seasoned with cumin, savory, Parkelp, adding a small amount of chicken stock. Serve on toasted points from 1 slice of low-calorie bread)		236 40	5 7
Herb tea or black coffee		0	0
		276	12

MID-MORNING			
Choice of herb tea, iced or hot. No sugar		0	0

LUNCH			
Fresh lean haddock or flounder, poached in stock or broiled (116-g. or 4½-oz. portion). Serve with lemon wedge		100	0
Large combination salad (Combine cold leftover vegetables with a few drops of salad oil, vinegar. Serve on lettuce strips)	1 generous cup	90 max.	5 approx.
Herb tea or demitasse		0	0
		190	5

MID-AFTERNOON	*Serving*	*Calories*	*CHO*
Tan, composed of ¾ cup plain yogurt, blended with water and chipped ice	Add ice, serve in tall glass	90	8 approx.

DINNER		*Calories*	*CHO*
Whole breast young chicken, roasted with capers, tarragon-style.		230	0
8 lightly steamed green asparagus spears OR ½ cup brussels sprouts, steamed		26	T
½ cup poached soybean sprouts OR 1 scant cup green string beans, poached		25	5 approx.
Small tossed salad (Mix a few drops oil and vinegar, a few fine sliced or diced scallions, chopped lettuce)		20	T
		301	5 T

MID-EVENING		*Calories*	*CHO*
Herb tea fizz		0	0

Day 10 Total Calories: 456 Carbohydrates: 15 g.

BREAKFAST	*Serving*	*Calories*	*CHO*
Hot lemonade (Pour ½ tsp. fresh lemon into 1 cup boiling water)	1 cup	0	0
1 boiled egg, sprinkled with tarragon, Parkelp		70	0
Tall glass herb tea, seltzer, chipped ice		0	0
		70	0

LUNCH

Chicken tan, a delight with a bonus (For four: two birds. Halve each, stuff many skin slits with bits of

	Serving	Calories	CHO
chopped onion. Marinate overnight in 1 cup light dry sherry with chopped onion cover. In A.M. add 1 pint natural yogurt, 1 tbsp. curry powder, 1 crushed garlic clove, ⅛ tsp. ground ginger, 1 tbsp. lime juice, 1 tbsp. melted butter. Mix. Marinate 2 hours more, or longer until brunch. Broil chicken with marinate, turning and basting. Allow 25 minutes each side, low to medium fire)	½ broiler *Have the gravy this time—it's counted! Entire portion	326*	4
Raw salad strips of green pepper, carrot slivers, cress, mint sprigs, diced fennel leaves, cucumber and celery slices. (We're not counting calories or CHO—this is a "free" salad for dieters who need a lift this tenth day. Roughage is high and quite probably necessarily so. Recipe for four is to encourage you to invite company, *work* at preparing, at cleaning house. "Free" salad is your reward. Eat plenty as guests have soup, appetizer, dessert, but you don't)	1 generous portion	"0"	"0"
Iced herb tea, hot tea or demitasse		0	0
		326	4

DINNER

	Serving	Calories	CHO
Hot consommé (Use fat-free chicken stock)	1 cup	0	0
Raw salad vegetables, as in lunch. If using leftovers, refrigerate until used. (Another "free" reward, calories not counted*)	equiv. 1 cup	"0"	"0"

**Make those "zero" calorie and CHO counts we have inserted as pick-me-up rewards to get you over the hump of the tenth day a reality by making a real effort to exercise the body. Don't sit this day out. Burn up those extras we believe you need to provide a clean sweep-down, as well as a lift.*

	Serving	*Calories*	*CHO*
Tall *tan* (Blend 2 tbsp. yogurt, ½ cup chicken stock, with fistful of leftover salad vegetables or your greens mix. Serve with pulp on chipped ice or cubes)	1 tall glass	20	1+
½ grapefruit OR ⅔ cup fresh ripe strawberries, no sugar on either		40	10 approx.
Herb tea or demitasse	1 cup	0	0
		60	11+

MID-EVENING

Hot blueberry leaf tea or your choice of unsweetened beverage	1 cup	0	0

Day 11 Total Calories: 739 Carbohydrates: 39.4 g.

BREAKFAST	*Serving*	*Calories*	*CHO*
Chilled fruit cup (Combine ½ peach, a slice of pear, a slice of apple, and a thin melon slice. Top with 3 blueberries OR 2 strawberries		46-47	10 approx.
Health nut yogurt (Mix 2 tbsp. yogurt, 2 almonds, 1 walnut, 1 tsp. sesame seeds, 10 alfalfa seed sprouts, a pinch of fresh wheat germ, sprinkles of fresh yeast powder and bonemeal. Top with a few anise, fennel or caraway seeds and sprinkles of ginger, clove and/or nutmeg)		30-32	4
Petmez or dark honey	1 tsp.	22*	6
Herb tea or black coffee	1 cup	0	0
		101	20 approx.

**This count is for honey*—petmez *is lower in calories.*

LUNCH	*Serving*	*Calories*	*CHO*
Broiled lule kabob (Lace a 3-oz. or 85-g. ball composed of leftover fine-ground lamb, veal, turkey, chicken or beef, in any mix, with 1 tbsp. finely chopped scallion and a mixture of green pepper, dill, parsley, oregano, thyme. To this, add ½ tsp. tomato puree and sprinkles of Parkelp, *chaimen* (ground fenugreek) or ground cumin seed, or dry mustard. Mix well and roll into a ball. Skewer, Broil a few minutes to taste)	1 kabob	150	2
Bulgur pilaf with sprouts (Cook 3 tbsp. *bulgur* wheat in fat-free chicken stock to absorb, adding a pinch of sprouted alfalfa when cooked)		48	10
Tossed green salad (Mix thin slices of onion, tomato, cucumber, dill and chopped lettuce to make the equivalent of 1 cup. Don't pack the cup)		45	6
Salad dressing (Mix well 1 scant tbsp. salad oil with 1 cubic in. or 17 g. of bleu or Roquefort cheese)		200	T
Herb tea, hot or iced		0	0
		443	18 T

DINNER			
Grilled filet of sole, 135 g. or 4¾ oz., raw		105	0
Fresh steamed crab salad (Combine ½ cup crabmeat, ¼ cup chicken stock, 10 drops Tabasco sauce, 1 tsp. grated onion, ¼ tsp. salad oil, ⅓ cup raw diced celery, ½ tsp. lemon, a sprinkle of dill, 1 tsp.			

	Serving	Calories	CHO
alfalfa sprouts, shredded lettuce. Steam crab in stock, drain, mix with other ingredients. Top with dill and alfalfa, using lettuce as bed. Chill)		90	1.4
Herb tea or demitasse		0	0
		195	1.4

MID-EVENING

	Serving	Calories	CHO
Herb tea fizz	1 tall glass	0	0

Day 12 Total Calories: 715 Carbohydrates: 37.5 g.

BREAKFAST	Serving	Calories	CHO
*Red and green cocktail (Blenderize selected greens as in Day 1 menu, add ½ cup tomato juice. Might vary by adding 5 drops Tabasco sauce, sprinkles of Parkelp, fennel, ground ginger, allspice and/or anise. Greens can be selected from raw Swiss chard, green fennel, chives, beet greens, shallots, scallions, onions, mustard greens, fresh turnip greens. Blend can be topped with sprinkle of fresh parsley)	1 tall glass, with ice	21 approx.	5 approx.
Liver and bacon daymaker (Braise a medium slice of Canadian			

**Note: In this and previous greens juice blends, the calorie–CHO counts will vary. In this one, the count assumes a total of ¼ cup combined chopped fennel, chive, shallots, scallions, onions, beet greens, mustard greens, chard and turnip greens. By averaging calories for 4 oz. of all but shallots (1 oz.), scallions and onions (2 oz. each), we come up with an average of 21 calories, more or less, and a scant 5 CHO, more or less. Ice and some water added to provide more liquid and lessen pulp taste add nothing. So we confess that our calorie–CHO counts in greens juices are approximate, subject to variance, depending on your formula. However, these juices are important to know, to drink often. By pushing some calories through unabsorbed, their fiber effects will certainly make up for any extra calories you may include.*

	Serving	*Calories*	*CHO*
bacon or 2 to 3 thin slices **basterma* or *soudjuk*. While dressing, soak a 37-g. or 1.4-oz. slice of calf or lamb liver in milk. To cook, drain, sprinkle with Parkelp, allspice, black pepper, finely chopped parsley. Pan broil, brushing pan with a speck of oil and garlic or onion rub. Brown liver 2 to 3 minutes total, both sides. Do not overcook)		190	3
Low-calorie bread	1 slice	40 max.	7 max.
Herb tea or black coffee	1 cup	0	0
		251	15 max.

LUNCH

Fruit cock-coction (Finely chop 2 slices raw zucchini, one 50-g. or 1¾-oz. cold, cooked beet, ¼ cup raw red raspberries, ½ cup ripe strawberries. Add 2 drops each of vanilla, almond and lemon extract. Use half of the above for lunch on shredded lettuce bed, saving rest to chill in flavorless gelatin and have on another day in place of approximately same number of calories/CHO as you may need to substitute)		45	10
Top either serving of above with 65 g. or 2.3 oz. of cottage cheese. If you have time to fuss a little, extrude cheese through pastry tube as a rim around the fruit		69	1.8 max.
Bonus: Further top with 1 tbsp. pressurized cream whip. Skip if you're a Spartan		10	T
Low-calorie bread	1 slice	40 max.	7 max.

**See Chapter 11 recipe.*

	Serving	Calories	CHO
38-g. or 1⅓-oz. wedge Camembert OR 30-g. or 1-oz. wedge bleu or brick cheese		115	1 max.
Herb tea or demitasse	1 cup	0	0
		279	20

DINNER

	Serving	Calories	CHO
Broiled filet of flounder or sole (90 g. or a scant 3 oz.)		105	0
Homemade cole slaw: ½ cup thinly sliced cabbage, well-mixed with a few drops French dressing or, if you must, a dab of mayonnaise		70	2.5 max.
Small salad of radish slices, cress, thin cucumber slices, chopped lettuce. No dressing tonight. Be Spartan. We're nearly home		10	T
Iced tea, herb tea or coffee	1 cup	0	0
		185	2.5

MID-EVENING

	Serving	Calories	CHO
Herb tea fizz	1 glass	0	0

Day 13 Total Calories: 730 Carbohydrates: 51-3 g.

BREAKFAST	Serving	Calories	CHO
½ breast of chicken (78 g. or 2¾ oz.) (Marinate the chicken overnight in grated onion, 6 ounces of white wine. Remove from marinate. Debone and sauté chicken in dab of butter and 1 tbsp. marinate. Poach 50 g. or 1¾ oz. fennel strips, quartered from base. Remove chicken before browned, then complete with fennel in skillet with 1 to 2 tbsp. stock. Allow 5 minutes, each side.			

	Serving	*Calories*	*CHO*
Top with 1 tbsp. whipped butter, 1 tbsp. half'n'half cream over both chicken and fennel)		200	2 T
Poached apple, rice pilaf (prepare night before. Quarter 1 small fresh apple. Poach 2 minutes in enough chicken stock to cover. Border apple with brown rice pilaf cooked in chicken stock. Heat before serving)		70	15
Your choice of a noncaloric beverage, hot or cold		0	0
		270	17 T
LUNCH			
Hot, steamed cauliflower buds (120 g. or 4½ oz.)	1 cup	25	3 max.
½ medium-sized melon with a generous scoop of cottage cheese, sprinkles of cayenne, nutmeg, Parkelp		184	25 T
Herb tea fizz	1 glass	0	0
		209	28
DINNER			
Grilled Canadian bacon (2 medium slices) OR equivalent in *basterma* or *soudjuk*		110	T
Serve above with 1 cup poached leek (110 g. or 3.88 oz.) and ½ cup poached zucchini (6 g. or 1/5 oz.)		66	7
Wedge of American cheese (18 g. or .6 oz.)		60	1
Small tossed green salad of endive, cress and lettuce, with cheese wedge above crumbed on as dressing		15	T
Herb tea or demitasse		0	0
		251	8 T

MID-EVENING	*Serving*	*Calories*	*CHO*
Herb tea fizz	1 glass	0	0

Day 14 Total Calories: 808 Carbohydrates: 42 g.

BREAKFAST	*Serving*	*Calories*	*CHO*
Trout, brook preferably, portion approximately 6″ long (120 g. or 4¼ oz.) (Marinate briefly in a few ounces of dry sherry, tarragon, chervil, Par-kelp sprinkles. Dip in half'n'half cream before placing in hot, buttered pan. Brown rapidly. Avoid burning)		121	0
Garnish fish with ½ tsp. chopped parsley, a few drops of lemon juice. In serving, pour remains of hot butter over fish. (Calorie count allows up to 1½ tbsp. whipped butter)		95	T
*Persimmon flambage. We know breakfast can be a rush but we're celebrating the last day of the diet. (Quarter one 123 g. or 4.4 oz. *ripe* persimmon, leaving it joined at the base. Pour 1 tsp. brandy on fruit and touch with match to light. Serve) (*Caution:* Use only ripe fruit or suffer unpleasant puckery taste)		95	20
Herb tea or black coffee	1 cup	0	0
		311	20 T

LUNCH			
Chicken stock consommé (Garnish with a pinch of alfalfa sprouts, top with 1 tbsp. yogurt)	1 cup	7	T

**If unavailable, substitute ¾ cup fresh pear slices or ¾ cup fresh diced peach.*

	Serving	Calories	CHO
Frivolitees (U.S. lamb fries) (Dip 2 halves lamb testicle (48 g. or 1¾ oz.) in milk and braise 2 minutes on each side in butter-brushed skillet) (You'll need butcher's cooperation in ordering the lamb fries)		60	T
Small tossed green salad, your choice of greens	½ cup	15	T
Herb tea or demitasse	1 cup	0	0
		82	1 max.

DINNER

	Calories	CHO
Filet mignon (111 g. or 4 oz., raw) (Flatten meat with whack of pan, brush with oil, broil under hot flame to taste—rare, medium or well. Just before serving, add a drop of soya sauce or Kitchen Bouquet. At table, splash with Burgundy wine and enflamme to celebrate last night of diet)	300	T
8 medium-sized Brussels sprouts, steamed, seasoned with summer savory	55	10
Baked potato, small- to medium-sized	60	10-11
Herb tea or demitasse	0	0
	415	20-21

MID-EVENING

	Calories	CHO
Herb tea fizz	0	0

Congratulations!

I know that, for many, some of our breakfasts have gone against habit and tradition. I also know many of these meals have been a chore to prepare. Dieters facing a morning rush have had to rise earlier and, often as not, do some of the work the night before. Diet lunches are always troublesome for those who must work—ours no less so than the others. But if you're serious about this effort and what it will accomplish for you, you'll find converts among fellow workers, the more the better to divide up the daily luncheon responsibility. If your office doesn't have a refrigerator, campaign for one or locate one nearby you can use. Trouble? Remember, health and longevity are worth any trouble.

Our diet and nutritional habits will lead to longevity, better health and better performance in and enjoyment of sex. That's the way of the Caucasus people, the most and best examples of longevity we have found on earth. Their secret is no secret at all but a way of living that has never turned away from nature to chemistry.

What I've outlined for you with strongest conviction is a way of life common among most of our ancestors until the 1840s when the big mills began processing, exposing limbs, hearts, lungs, stomachs and blood vessels—conditioned by centuries to food from nature —to synthetic feeds, processed and chemicalized more and more as the years have passed.

One very palatable way to end that diet is in the next, and final, chapter of our book. It's a great personal pleasure to introduce now Barbara Apisson's recipes for Caucasus-style cookery of American and other favorites.

11.

Blessings From Barbara

Barbara Apisson's cooking style combines excellent taste results with the healthy nutrition habits Dr. Williams recommends for better health and longer years.* All recipes are for four unless otherwise stated. By following quantity instructions carefully and by adopting the entire spectrum of health habits the doctor has suggested, such as serious exercise, most of you will have to work hard to defeat these meals and gain weight on them.

Arithmetic will be needed to cook for more or less than four. Obviously, these meals will do the most for healthy people. They are not meant as substitutes for medical treatment for sick people. Chronic weight gainers will find more to benefit them in Chapter 10 than in Barbara's meals. Some may find a way out by dividing their efforts more or less evenly between the two chapters. The results you obtain by experimenting with both chapters will guide you to a regimen that works best for you. For most who are overweight, switching back and forth, as may be necessary, will provide a long-term downturn to healthier weight levels. Once at ideal weight, for most readers these meals and a rising program of exercise will provide weight maintenance and longer years.

Caucasus recipes, particularly those mentioned earlier by Dr. Williams, have been included. But as we have indicated, these are not so much Caucasus recipes as Barbara Apisson's Caucasus ways of preparing American dishes.

Barbara's husband, Henri Apisson, tells his diners, "Every-

**Ed. Note: Here Dr. Williams is no longer providing the notes. This portion of the book has been developed with Barbara Apisson, by interview; also from handwritten recipes.*

thing at West Point Farms is made with love. But how much love—that is our secret." Thousands of diners have wondered how Barbara Apisson does it. These are her secrets, revealed for the first time.

CHICKEN STOCK

Barbara deploys her chicken and fish stocks and concentrates so lavishly that it would be impossible to start you on her style of cooking without the recipes for all three. Her chicken stock recipe makes five to six quarts. When the supply gets low, the leftover stock is the number one ingredient for starting a new batch. In any health-oriented kitchen, as in Barbara's, stock is forever.

Ingredients: 2 large hens with a total combined weight of 7 to 8 lbs.; 1 cup white cooking wine OR 2 to 3 tbsp. vinegar; 3 celery stalks with their leaves; 1 medium carrot; 1 medium sweet onion; 1 leek with its greens; ½ parsnip (optional); ¼ bunch parsley; 5 to 6 egg whites, one for each quart. (Use the entire hen, diverting only the liver. But don't discard the liver. As you read earlier, it is excellent food. Use it in some other way. Everything else edible—stomach, heart and feet included—is useful in stock.)

Place the two whole hens in a soup pot with enough water to cover. Next time, start with leftover stock and add enough extra water to cover. Simmer for 2 hours. Add wine or vinegar. Wine provides a better taste, but vinegar is good because it releases calcium from the bones. Next add the vegetables, cut up as you like them, in the soup. Cook for 1 more hour.

Chill until fat solidifies on top. Remove all fat. Beat the egg whites slightly with a fork and stir into the cold stock. Place over a low heat and stir. When stock starts simmering, stop stirring. The egg whites should now have coagulated, gathering into their mass all the bits which make the stock cloudy.

Allow ten minutes for this process. Remove the stock from the heat and strain through double cheesecloth. What remains is clear stock ready for use.

Do not discard the leftovers in the cheesecloth. If you have animals, feed them the mix, removing all bones. If you have no other use in mind, the mash—bones and all—makes fine garden food. Give it directly to the earth or to your compost heap.

Refrigerate the stock between uses. If it is not used up in two weeks, reboil, cool, refrigerate again and continue to use it until it is gone or disappears into your next batch of stock.

Don't worry about calories in this fat-free stock. Learn to use it in cooking operations in which you presently use water. You saw its use in the diet meals. It is just as valuable in the recipes ahead.

CONCENTRATE

Once every two weeks to a month or so, depending on how many ways you learn to use it, you'll want to prepare concentrate, another basic in Barbara's cuisine.

Ingredients: 4 lbs. of beef bones with meat still on them (you may prefer that amount of veal—or, if you like, you may use roughly equal quantities of beef and veal bones with meat on them); 1 cup white table wine; 3 tbsp. natural apple-cider vinegar; 2 whole onions; 3 celery stalks, including the leaves; ½ bunch parsley.

Combine all ingredients in enough water to cover the meat and cook on a high heat until simmering. Lower the heat and allow to simmer on a low flame for 5 hours. (If you wish, add more meat, off the bone, at this time—2 to 3 lbs. more will help the concentrate and contribute to a good meal when removed.) Cook 1 hour or longer, as necessary, to tenderize the meat. Let it cool. Remove the meat and bones for other uses. Strain. Refrigerate. When fat solidifies on top, skim off all of it.

Replace the pot on a high heat. Boil the stock down until it is syrupy. You may want to use a stovetop plate to avoid burning at this point. You will have to stir continually toward the end. When very thick, remove from the fire. Cool the stock for a short time and then pour into coverable jars. Refrigerate when cool enough. Keeps two weeks.

Reheat the concentrate when needed. It will not sour. If it's kept longer than two weeks, simmer again and store in the refrigerator until used. Barbara's rule: Never run out of stock; never run out of concentrate. Can you use the commercial products on the market? We don't recommend any with additives, especially those with monosodium glutamate. When concentrate runs low, as with stock, use leftovers to start your next batch.

SAUCE

This gourmet roast enhancer will earn the chef family hurrahs. Mix ½ cup concentrate with ½ cup dry wine. (For large roasts, use 1 cup concentrate, 1 cup wine. For lamb or beef, use red wine; for turkey or veal, use white. Any table wine will do.) Simmer ½ hour over medium heat. This will reduce the amount of your mix by 50 percent. After the roast is prepared (see our instructions for roasts), heat the sauce and add as garnish when serving.

FISH STOCK

This recipe makes two quarts. Unlike chicken stock, leftover fish stock cannot be used to start the next batch. Plan to consume fish stock in a week and then make more from scratch. If little fish is used in your home, halve the recipe until that bad habit is overcome and make fish stock only when you know you are going to use it. At West Point Farms, there is always fish stock, just as there is always chicken stock and concentrate, on hand.

Ingredients: ½ large chopped onion; enough fresh parsley, chopped with its stem, to fill 1 tbsp.; 2 lbs. whiting with the bones and trimmings, as well as the bones and trimmings of one sole (you'll use sole filets for a meal, of course); juice of ½ lemon; 2 to 3 pints water; 1 cup white wine.

Blanch the onions and parsley for 2 to 3 minutes in a pot. Add fish, bones and all the trimmings. Add lemon juice. Simmer for 5 minutes or so, shaking the pot at intervals to move the ingredients around. Add 1½ quarts (3 pints) of water. Bring to a boil. Skim off brownish foam that settles on top. Simmer 15 minutes longer. Add wine and simmer again for 15 minutes. Strain the stock through a colander, forcing as much whiting through as possible. Any small bone particles that get through are good for you. Cool and refrigerate. Use what's left in the colander in your garden. Barbara does.

FISH SAUCE

Ingredients: 1 chopped onion; 1 or 2 garlic cloves, peeled and crushed; 1 celery stalk, chopped; 2 tbsp. chopped parsley; ½ cup vegetable oil; 1 tsp. oregano; 1 lb. chopped tomatoes; 1 cup fish stock. (Oregano is dried, but best fresh if available. It seldom is.)

Sauté the onion, garlic, celery and parsley in vegetable oil. When tender, add the oregano and tomatoes. Simmer for ½ hour. Add the fish stock. Simmer for 10 minutes more. Use immediately or refrigerate when cool for later use.

Reminder: Barbara mixes her cooking oils for general cooking—⅓ each of safflower, sunflower and corn, omitting soya, except for special purposes, and omitting peanut because she feels its flavor is too pervasive. Re-read in Chapter 4 about vitamin F if you have forgotten why Barbara and Dr. Williams prefer this mix. In all of Barbara's recipes, when she calls for oil, this mix is preferred, but you may have your own all-vegetable favorite. Experiment a bit with oils.

TOMATO SAUCE

Ingredients: 2 lbs. peeled, chopped fresh tomatoes or a 16-oz. can of peeled Italian tomatoes with no preservatives; 1 large chopped onion; 2 to 3 chopped garlic cloves; 1 medium chopped green pepper; ½ bunch of chopped parsley; 1 finely chopped tender celery stalk with the leaves; 1 tbsp. whole-wheat flour; 1 tsp. oregano; ½ tsp. rosemary; 1 tsp. basil; 4 tbsp. vegetable oil; ½ tsp. *petmez* (or 1 tsp. dark honey); ½ cup white wine if tomatoes are fresh or 1 cup if canned; salt and pepper to taste. (If canned tomatoes are packed with no tomato paste, add 1 tbsp. of tomato paste.)

Sauté all solid ingredients in oil for 10 minutes. Add *petmez* (or honey). Add wine. Stir gently for 2 to 3 minutes. If tomato paste is used, add it now. Simmer on a low flame for 30 minutes more. Salt and pepper just before removing from fire.

DILL SAUCE

Topping for vegetables, salad, fish or leftovers.
Ingredients: 4 egg yolks; 1 tsp. fresh dill; 1 tsp. dark honey (or somewhat less *petmez*); juice of ½ lemon, or 1 tsp. apple-cider vinegar; 2 tsp. arrowroot powder; 3 cups of stock. Use chicken stock for vegetables. Use fish stock for topping for fish or seafood.

Beat the egg yolks. Add the dill, honey (or *petmez*), lemon or vinegar. Now add arrowroot to the cold stock and heat but do not boil. Pour thickened stock into egg mix. Heat slowly. Remove from the fire when nearing a boil. Use hot or cold.

TAHINI DRESSING

Used with fish, shellfish, chick-peas or vegetables.
Ingredients: 2 tbsp. *tahini* (sesame paste); 2 tbsp. oil; 2 tbsp. lemon juice; 1 clove of garlic squeezed through garlic press.

Combine ingredients and mix thoroughly. Use a blender if you like your dressings smooth. Good on hot or cold dishes, those indicated or your choice.

GIBLET GRAVY (Not for dieters)

Ingredients: Giblets of one turkey or two chickens; chicken stock to cover; 1 cup sweet cream or half n'half cream; ½ cup white wine.

Use all turkey or chicken giblets except the liver. Include feet if available. Cover the giblets with stock and boil. Lower the flame. Simmer for 1 hour, or until tender. Cool. Bone out the neck meat, then slice up the heart and stomach. Put giblet meats into blender and add enough of your cooked stock to cover. Purée. Add remaining stock, and mix in the sweet cream or half n'half. Add the white wine. Stir gently. Simmer for 5 minutes. The gravy is now ready to use. A hint to improve it: If you have roasted fowl, skim out the glaze, chill and skim off fat. Add what's left to your giblet gravy.

ARMENIAN SOUL FOOD

A heavenly "biscuit" mix, this nutritious pastry is a base for chop-chop (see recipe in "Breakfasttime") and can be used for any number of equally good purposes. Barbara Apisson simply calls this "cheese," but we named it to give it its own identity, because everything she tops this blissful basic with is celestial—pâtés, spreads, hors d'oeuvres, dips. It is a fine high-protein "pastry" base.

Ingredients: ½ lb. sharp, hard cheese (Barbara prefers Swiss); ½ lb. feta cheese; ½ cup vegetable oil; 1 cup whole-wheat flour; 1 egg; a dash of paprika. (You'll have to multiply the recipe if preparing for crowds.)

Grate the hard cheese, crumble the feta, mix the cheeses and add all but 4 to 5 tbsp. of the mix to the oil. Sift in flour and mix well. Place the mass on a piece of wax paper and refrigerate until firm enough to roll out, as for biscuits. Roll to a flat sheet between ¼" and ½" thick, no more. Place on an unbuttered cookie sheet. If you are making hors d'oeuvres, cut into squares 1½ x 1½". If making chop-chop or a variant, bake uncut.

Stir the egg with a fork until beaten and brush over the top of the dough. Sprinkle on remaining grated or crumbled cheese. Dust with paprika. Bake for 20 minutes in a preheated 350°F. oven.

Once you get the hang of Armenian soul food, family and friends will hail this base for all your favorite spreads, avoiding bases that call for white flour. Chop-chop is one example of a spread for this base which we'll be giving you in this chapter.

YOGURT (*MADZOON*) #1

To make good yogurt, it is important to start with a good commercial plain yogurt or a starter supply from a recipe you know and like. Once you have your own, use it to make your next batch. Prepare or cool in pyrex or glass. Test temperatures with a cooking thermometer.

Ingredients: 1 quart whole milk; ¼ cup plain yogurt.

Bring milk close to a boil (200°F.) over a medium low heat. If skim forms, do not remove it. Remove pot from heat. Cool to 120°F. Pour 4 tbsp. warm milk into yogurt in a mixing bowl and mix until well blended. Pour the mix back into the milk. Stir gently to work it in. Set out of a draft—in the oven, for instance—the top protected by heavy towel, and maintain a 110°F. temperature for 4 to 5 hours. (If the mix cools, apply a little heat to get it back up to 110°F.) The mix should thicken in that time. Refrigerate and use as you prefer or in our recipes. You'll find many uses for yogurt on these pages.

ANOTHER YOGURT (Not for dieters) #2

As you read earlier, yogurt is a wonderful food. Be patient if its taste is tart and new. You'll learn to enjoy that taste without sweeteners. That's the way it's best for you. This recipe makes twice as much and is higher in calories because of the cream.

Ingredients: 2 quarts whole milk; 8 tbsp. heavy cream; 8 tbsp. plain yogurt.

Bring milk to 200 °F., as above. Mix the cream and yogurt well, stir into milk and let stand at 110°F., protected as shown above. When it's thick (4 to 5 hours), cool and refrigerate.

STILL ANOTHER (Not for dieters) #3

Ingredients: 2 quarts certified raw milk; 8 tbsp. heavy cream; 8 tbsp. plain yogurt.

Heat the milk to 110°F. Stir in the yogurt–cream mix as in the recipe above and keep the mix protected at 90–100°F. for 4 to 5 hours. When thick, cool and refrigerate.

YOGURT DRESSING (Non-dieters only)

Use this dressing instead of sour cream or mayonnaise. It's much healthier. Once accustomed to the taste, you'll prefer and flourish on it.

Ingredients: 1 pint whole milk; 1 pint heavy cream; ¼ cup plain yogurt. Follow directions in #1 above for preparing. If the heavy cream worries you, remember that yogurt culturing pre-digests the cream, giving you a utility different from heavy cream, sour cream or whole milk.

In the Caucasus and elsewhere, people who can't tolerate milk and cream benefit from yogurt, without milk or cream discomfort, as a palatable source of all those yogurt nutrients you saw listed in our earlier chapters.

That's our group of basic items you'll need to provide ingredients for recipes to come and for extra pleasure and rewards in cooking as you begin to improvise in the creation of your own healthful, nutritious dishes, avoiding less beneficial stocks, sauces, gravies and dressings you may have used in the past.

BREAKFASTTIME

Our Dr. Williams is among the medical people who endorse a hearty breakfast. Nothing is more logical. Bodies normally go the longest without food from dinnertime to breakfasttime. We need ample nourishment more when we wake than at any other time.

People who rush off with lick-and-promise breakfasts take on their morning's work nutritionally unprepared. Caucasus farmers never dream of breakfasting that way. It makes as little sense for the rest of us.

If you must eat lightly, do it at lunch. Midday, one should not have so much food as to occupy the body so with digestion that the mind dulls for afternoon work. Lunch should be just enough to tide you over until dinner. Breakfast and dinner should be the day's large meals. You need nothing in between unless you are on a prescribed many-snack routine. Little if anything is needed for TV watching after dinner.

As Dr. Williams told you, proteins are the foods that most satisfy our needs. Barbara's girlhood in the Caucasus blossomed on big protein-rich breakfasts.

Organ meats, with or without eggs, deserve to be more popular for breakfast than they are in America. Cattle-country breakfast steaks are common. The intention is good, but the meat is wrong. If steak *is* used, it should be lean. Organ meats are better as day starters. They walk us away from saturated fats as they provide protein. Our way of serving organ meats for breakfast (and at other times) is chop-chop.

Since closing the inn part of West Point Farms, Barbara no longer serves breakfast to the public. The Apissons begin their own breakfasts not with sweetened frozen juices but with whole fresh fruit, sometimes stewed fruit topped with yogurt, oranges, prunes, figs, pears, apples, whatever. Readers should switch to fresh or home-stewed fruit, too. After your fruit, breakfast should emphasize proteins.

As you have read, whole-grain cereals are rich in protein. So are eggs. There are many sources of breakfast proteins. In place of processed breakfast meats you are accustomed to, try chop-chop with its organ meats. Make the ingredients the night before, refrigerate and bake just before serving.

Eggs should be used sparingly by some, not at all by others. For extra protein, they can be served as liver, kidney, tripe, brain or sweetbread omelettes. You can mix two or more of these ad lib, as you'll see done in chop-chop.

Lamb fries (remember those wife-hunting Caucasus centenarians?), which Dr. Williams brought up several times, offer fine protein and taste values when available. You may have to be very specific with your butcher as to what they are. Barbara's recipe appears later. A diet preparation of this dish is in the final luncheon of Chapter 10.

Cheese is a fine breakfast-protein food. Eat it with whole-grain bread and black or green olives. Learn to like more cheeses. Experiment. Buy new ones when they are on sale. An international taste in cheeses is a healthy way of life, breakfast or whenever.

Yogurt is a perfect breakfast food because of the many values you have seen in our lists, including protein and calcium. It is truly super-food. Half a cup of homemade yogurt or a good plain commercial brand (skip the sugary fruit flavors you absolutely don't need) with soaked, dried mulberries added when you can get them; or soaked dried raisins or apricots, sulfur-free; or sliced fresh fruits in season, is a wonderful day starter.

Rennet custard (*saleb* to Caucasus people) is good breakfast food that can be prepared in advance.

Combine any of these suggestions within reason. A good

breakfast followed by an active day will be burned up. Not so a heavy lunch followed by a heavy dinner followed by an evening of heavy TV watching and snacking.

Compose original common-sense breakfasts by this philosophy, emphasizing proteins. As a starter, here are recipes to add to yours for nutrition and variety.

Chop-Chop

This is Barbara Apisson's topping (there can be many) for Armenian soul food. It's an exciting breakfast food, good for any meal or as a snack. With the soul food sheet rolled out, uncut as per earlier instructions, top with chop-chop before baking.

Ingredients: 1 lamb kidney or its equivalent; about 1 tbsp. of veal kidney; about 3 tbsp. of beef, chicken, lamb or pork liver, as you prefer; the equivalent of 2 tsp. veal heart; a more or less equal amount (to all the above) of the leanest mixed chopped beef and lamb you can find; 1 clove garlic; ½ green pepper; 1 medium onion or scallion; 1 medium tomato; 1 tbsp. yogurt; 1 tsp. basil; ½ tsp. paprika. Grind all organ meats together with the beef and lamb. Mix vigorously by hand until well blended. Chop the garlic, pepper, onion and tomato very fine, mix, add yogurt and stir with meat mix. Add basil and paprika. Mix well, salt and pepper to taste, but try to reduce salt if you are a heavy user.

Spread this mix evenly over the soul food base on cookie sheet or pie tin. Bake in a 350°F. oven for 20 minutes, as indicated in soul food recipe. Serve hot for breakfast, snacks, hors d'oeuvres or any meal you like.

***Tarama*'n'Eggs**

Ingredients: 6 eggs; 2 tbsp. hot water; a dab of butter; 1 tbsp. finely chopped chives; 2 tbsp. pink *tarama* (roe); 2 tbsp. yogurt.

Separate the eggs. Beat the yolks and add hot water when the color lightens. Beat the whites stiff and fold into the yolks. Butter and heat an omelette pan and then spoon in the eggs. Cook over a low flame until the omelette rises and sets. Put under the broiler long enough to brown. Mix the chives and *tarama.* Add the yogurt. Spread this mix on half the omelette. Turn the uncovered half over on your mix, brown in the oven and it's done.

Tomato Omelette

Ingredients: 6 eggs; 2 tbsp. hot water; a dab of butter for the omelette; 4 medium tomatoes, skinned and chopped; 1 tbsp. chopped fresh parsley; 1 tsp. vegetable oil; and pinches of salt and pepper.

Prepare the omelette as in *tamara*'n'eggs above. Sauté tomatoes and parsley in vegetable oil until tender. Pour the mix over half the omelette. Turn the other half over it, brown and serve.

A shortcut method for one: skin and slice 1 medium tomato, sauté in vegetable oil until tender. Beat 1 egg, add ½ tsp. chopped parsley, and salt and pepper to taste. Pour the beaten egg over the sautéed tomato, cover, and cook over a low flame for 3 to 5 minutes. Serve. As a variation: slice ½ pepper julienne; sauté with the tomato. Proceed with the short or long method explained above.

Yogurt Oatmeal
An excellent breakfast cereal!
Ingredients: 2 cups plain yogurt; 1 egg; 1 tbsp. whole-wheat flour; ½ cup of oatmeal. Don't use quick or instant oats—or water in this recipe. Mix the yogurt, egg and flour well, bring to a boil on a low heat, add the oatmeal and bring to a boil again. Cook for 5 minutes over a low flame, stirring occasionally. Options: Season with butter, one pat or less per person, depending on diet. Add 1 to 2 tsp. bran and/or 1 tsp. raw wheat germ per person. At West Point Farms, Barbara adds a pat of butter and both bran and wheat germ.

Millet Cereal
Cook 1 pint milk with ½ cup hulled millet meal on a low flame or in a double-boiler for 15 minutes. (Millet cereal can be cooked the night before, reheating and adding milk as needed, mixing well.) Butter and season to taste and to diet. Learn to brush with butter. For your health, avoid drowning with butter. Yogurt makes a fine nutritious topping instead of butter once you're used to it. Barbara Apisson uses yogurt lavishly in these and other ways.

Cracked Wheat Cereal
Cook 1 pint chicken stock with ½ cup finely ground cracked wheat for 30 minutes. Season to taste.

This can be prepared the night before.

Sardines and Eggs
Get used to this high-protein breakfast and you'll enjoy it again and again.
Ingredients: 1 large tomato cut into 4 round slices; 4 eggs; 1 tbsp. vegetable oil; 1 small can of sardines (usually about 4 oz.); sprigs of parsley for garnish; salt and pepper to taste (remember, sardines are usually well-salted!).

Place 4 tomato slices in a casserole, carefully break an egg over each, dot each with vegetable oil, and top each with a sardine.

Bake for 20 minutes in a 325°F. oven, brown under broiler flame, garnish with parsley, salt, pepper and serve.

Baked Eggs'n'Cheese
Ingredients: ½ lb. cheese (American, young American, muenster or a mix of soft cheeses); ½ tsp. paprika; ½ tsp. cumin powder; ½ cup yogurt; 8 eggs.

The original is made with feta cheese. Americans will prefer cheeses they know better but may want to experiment by adding a bit of feta to others until they learn to like it. Half your cheese(s) should be slices, the other half grated or simply crumbled.

Cover the bottom of a casserole with the cheese slices. Mix the paprika and cumin into the yogurt. Use about half the yogurt mix to cover the cheese slices, spreading evenly. Break the eggs over this, and top with the remaining (crumbled) cheese pieces and yogurt. Bake for about 15 minutes in a 325°F. oven until the eggs are cooked and the cheese is melted in. Brown a bit under the flame if you like, but don't overdo. Serve right out of the oven.

Whole fruit, cereal or eggs, chop-chop as an occasional substitute as an organ meat day starter, with herbal teas or coffee—these items make fine breakfasts. If you prefer toast and cheese, use whole-grain breads. And read your labels. Avoid whole-grain breads that admit to processed white flour as an ingredient, or the addition of coloring without giving you any idea of how much is used—a fairly sure indication that you are getting disguised white bread. We prefer warming the bread, wrapped in foil. Toasting, as you have read, wastes food values.

Now let's talk a bit about lunch and what people should try to have in it.

LUNCHTIMES

Too many Americans who call themselves health-minded have a cup of commercial yogurt for lunch and feel they've dined prudently. To Barbara and Dr. Williams, a cup of yogurt (without the sugary fruit), a piece of fruit or a snack of cheese is an excellent item for active people to have as a between-meals bite. But even with all its fine values, yogurt is not by itself a balanced meal. It's not enough for lunch, nor, by itself, breakfast.

Before saying what does make up a balanced light lunch,

let's say what doesn't. A tablespoon or so of cottage cheese on either fresh or canned fruit salad, overbalanced toward calories and carbohydrates, is not a good lunch. A generous mound of cottage cheese on a bed of green lettuce or mixed greens (which are eaten, not left) eaten with a slice of genuine whole-grain bread lightly buttered, one piece of fresh fruit and a beverage like buttermilk, *tan, kefir* OR yogurt makes a fine balanced lunch. Dieters can use herbal tea as their beverage—for instance, peppermint tea, a fine digestant.

Barbara and Dr. Williams would oppose even such a lunch every day or frequently. Lunch, like breakfast and dinner, should vary. Even nutritious food is hard to balance completely. Effective balance is best achieved by running the gamut in menus.

What about sandwiches for lunch? Fine, if composed of whole-grain, whole-wheat or an authentic pumpernickel bread, fresh meats (not processed kinds) or fresh salad items, with plenty of good green lettuce, cole slaw or greens on the side.

Salad plates are excellent for lunch. Caesar salads or chef salads that combine protein (meats and cheeses) with greens are excellent, provided they are not drowned in high-calorie dressings and the good greens not all left behind in the bowl. Such a salad with one slice of whole-grain bread, one of the suggested beverages and no dessert is a good lunch. Dessert should simply not be a part of a light lunch. It adds the wrong values at the expense of the right ones.

Soup? If you follow our suggestions for lunch, you won't need it. But as part of your plan to vary your luncheons, a wholesome fresh vegetable soup or beef vegetable soup, plus a few slices of any cold, unprocessed meat, some greens and your beverage make a good change of pace.

In indicating what constitutes a balanced light-luncheon meal, we should stress that our reasoning applies even more vigorously to skipping lunch, or any meal, altogether. People who skip meals pay themselves back when their bodies demand it, usually the wrong way. The items that spring most quickly into your hands when you skip meals are candy bars, cakes, buns, muffins and similar offenders of balance—the junk foods. To avoid such required "rewards," don't skip meals. You owe yourself that much. If you must miss a meal, purposefully compensate with proteins, grains and greens as make-up snacks. Less fun? More health.

When we come to dinner recipes, remember that meat loaf, roasts, fish, fowl—all those good protein sources—make excellent leftovers for luncheons. Clever planning of dinners provides those protein sources cold for luncheons. When you don't need to buy your lunch, build it on wholesome protein leftovers you trust because you cooked them yourself. Why cold? Reheating usually means overbaking, overcooking, overroasting and sacrificing nutrients.

The next groupings all come under the heading of dinner items, but any of them may, Sundays or other special days, be a means of enjoying fine balanced luncheons, too. Just remember that lunch is a light meal. If you plan a big holiday lunch, fine. But dinner should be light that night. Or, since a heavier dinner tides everyone over to the following morning in better shape, why not make it a habit to invite guests for dinner instead of midday with that in mind?

Cheese *Beurek*

People not native to Middle Eastern countries who have had *beurek* elsewhere are never prepared for the mouth-watering experience of Barbara's. With regular diners at West Point Farms, beginning with anything but *beurek* is unthinkable.

Barbara developed this recipe after many early diners at her restaurant refused the traditional *beurek* made with feta and cottage cheese. The recipe we give you makes a dozen *beureks.* A family of four will consume those within a week and clamor for more. Barbara prepares larger batches in advance, refrigerates them (never longer than a week) and pops them into the oven to order.

To make the twelve, you'll need two dozen 10 x 12″ pieces of paper-thin commercial sheet dough if you want to buy dough ready-made. Greek food stores sell it as *filo.* Homemade sheet dough is always thicker than the commercial product, so you'll need only a dozen of the homemade for a dozen *beurek.* Let's start with the recipe for the sheet dough.

The Sheet Dough

This recipe makes some three dozen sheets, more or less, depending on how thin you roll them out. If a dozen are used to make *beurek,* the rest can be frozen indefinitely until needed for more *beureks,* or to make *bourmas* (see "Desserts"), or for anything else you want to make using paper-thin dough.

Ingredients: 1 egg; 2 tbsp. yogurt; ½ cup water; ½ tsp. salt; 2 tbsp. safflower oil; 2½ cups unbleached flour; 1 cup arrowroot, using as little at a time as necessary to roll out and separate layers of dough.

Mix the egg with a fork. Add yogurt, water, salt, oil. As you blend these ingredients together, slowly stir in the flour, working on a large breadboard or clean table surface lightly sprinkled with arrowroot. Knead to medium-soft dough consistency. Divide into a dozen equal dough balls. Lightly sprinkle arrowroot on the surface of the cookie sheet. Arrange the dough balls on the sheet and let them stand for 2 to 3 hours, covered with a faintly damp kitchen towel.

Spread a fresh sprinkling of arrowroot on the breadboard. Sprinkle also the surface of your rolling pin and a clean rounded stick (1½″ dowel) one yard in length which you should make and keep clean for this purpose.

Take each dough ball one at a time and roll flat to a circle about 10″ in diameter. Stack these dough circles three deep, sprinkling with arrowroot to keep them separated. A dozen dough balls will give you four round stacks of three.

Now roll each stack out thinner, first with the rolling pin, then with the dowel stick, until each stack of three has been flattened and extended to 10 x 36″ oblong. Now cut each stack into thirds, 10 x 12″ each. When you have rolled out and cut all four stacks of three, you should wind up with thirty-six 10 x 12″ oblong pieces. Use one dozen to make cheese *beureks* and freeze the rest for later use.

Cheese Mix for *Beurek*

Ingredients: 1 dozen homemade paper-thin dough sheets prepared as above or 2 dozen if purchased ready-made as *filo;* ½ cup butter; ½ cup safflower oil; 1 egg; 1 tsp. chopped parsley; ¼ lb. (or 4 oz.) muenster cheese; ⅛ lb. (or 2 oz.) Swiss cheese; ⅛ lb. feta cheese; ⅛ lb. young (white) American cheese. (These are the cheeses Barbara finally settled on for her *beurek.* Try it exactly this way and you'll discover what thousands have at West Point Farms.)

Set a single 10 x 12″ dough sheet (two thicknesses together if ready-made from store) on wax paper. Melt the butter. Add the safflower oil to the butter and mix. Use this mix to brush the dough surface lightly with a pastry brush. Beat the egg with a fork. Add parsley. Grate all cheeses into this mixture. Stir until well mixed. Put 2 heaping tbsp. of the cheese mix on the dough sheet, left of center. Position the cheese mix to permit folding one-third of the way across the 10″ width (3⅓″), covering the cheese. Then fold once more from left to right, so that you have double-folded the dough sheet into a package 3⅓″ wide and 12″ long.

This package is now folded up from the bottom to become a triangle. Make approximately equal folds from the lower right corner across to the left, and then fold up straight across, once more up and across from left to right and finally across and straight up. Tuck in any leftover dough to make an even triangle. When you've done it twelve times, your dozen *beureks* (if you make all at once) are ready to bake. Otherwise refrigerate those you want to save until later.

Assemble the *beureks* in a baking pan, brushing the outer

tops of all to be baked with oil/butter mix. Preheat your oven to 350°F. Bake for 20 minutes. Brown briefly under flame. Remove from oven. *Serve immediately.* If allowed to cool before eating, the cheese becomes rubbery, loses taste and disappoints. Like everything at West Point Farms, *beurek* is made to order, served piping hot. Dining there is leisurely, but *beurek* is best eaten immediately.

Lentil Soy Soup with *Tahini*

This is a nutrition feast.

Ingredients: ½ cup soybeans; ½ cup chick-peas; 1 cup pink lentils; 4 cups water; 4 cups chicken stock; 1 carrot; 2 celery stalks; 1 tbsp. chopped green pepper; 1 large onion; 3 tbsp. butter; 2 tsp. basil; 3 tbsp. chopped parsley; 2 tbsp. *tahini* (sesame paste).

Soak soybeans and chick-peas overnight to soften. For mineral values, save 4 cups water when you drain. Cook soybeans, lentils and chick-peas in stock and 4 cups water for 1 hour, or longer if necessary to tenderize. Cut up the carrot and celery and add along with the chopped pepper. Chop the onion fine and sauté it in butter with the basil, parsley and *tahini* until the color is pink. This takes about 5 minutes. When pink, add to soup and serve.

Yogurt Soup (*Tanabour*)

Ingredients: 3 cups chicken stock; ½ cup millet meal; 1 egg; 3 cups yogurt; 1 tsp. whole-wheat flour; ½ cup chopped onion; 3 level tsp. butter or 3 tbsp. vegetable oil; 1 tbsp. basil.

Warm the stock. Add the millet and simmer and until tender (15 to 20 minutes). Beat the egg into the yogurt and sift in the flour over a low heat. Stir constantly until it comes to a boil and immediately add to the cooking stock and millet. Brown the chopped onions in butter or oil. When browned, add basil, mix and pour into soup. Serve hot. For variations, substitute oatmeal or noodles for the ½ cup of millet.

Yogurt Nut Soup

Ingredients: 3 cups chicken broth; 2 tbsp. butter; 1 tbsp. millet meal; a pinch of ground cloves; a pinch of ground mace; 1 cup very finely chopped almonds; 2 pinches of ground thyme; 1 clove garlic; 1 tsp. paprika; ¼ tsp. cumin; a pinch of cayenne pepper; 1 cup yogurt; 2 tbsp. cooking sherry.

Warm the chicken stock. Melt the butter, mix in the millet meal and add to the stock. Mix and add all dry ingredients except for the cayenne pepper. Add the pepper to the yogurt and add both this and the wine just before serving. Yogurt nut soup cooks in about 30 minutes.

As with yogurt soup, you may vary this recipe by substituting for the millet an equal amount of noodles (whole-wheat) or oatmeal.

Vegetarian Vegetable Soup Purée

Ingredients: 1 medium celery root; 1 large parsley root; 1 large onion; 2 cloves garlic; 2 stalks celery with leaves; 2 tbsp. of fresh parsley chopped with the stems; 2 bay leaves; 1 tsp. rosemary leaves; 1 large potato; ½ tsp. fennel.

Chop all ingredients together, not too finely. Put all in a soup pot and add enough water to cover. Cook for 1 hour and strain entire contents of pot through Foley food mill or press through food sieve or strainer. Serves 4 to 5 persons. Serve hot.

Mongol Split Pea Soup

Ingredients: 2 cups chicken stock; ½ lb. yellow (mongol) split peas, purchased dried; 1 tbsp. chopped parsley; 2 cups whole milk; 2 tbsp. tomato paste; 1 tbsp. soy flour; 1 tsp. basil; and a pinch of nutmeg.

Put the stock, split peas and parsley in a soup pot and cook for 1 hour. Mix the milk, tomato paste, soy flour, add basil and sprinkle in nutmeg. Add all to soup. Simmer for 12 minutes more and serve. If the family prefers its pea soup thick enough to attack with a knife more or less, add ½ cup to 1 cup of concentrate to the stock at the beginning.

Vegetable Marrow Bone Soup

Ingredients: 2 beef marrow bones cut for soup; 3 lbs. veal bones with meat on them, cut into soup/meat portions for you by butcher from 3 legs of veal; 2 tbsp. vegetable oil; 2 cloves garlic; 1 large chopped onion; 2 stalks celery, chopped with leaves; 2 chopped med. carrots; 2 large tomatoes, chopped; 3 cups chicken stock; 3 cups water; pepper to taste; and 2 bay leaves (optional). (If you prefer, you may vary this soup by using all veal bones and veal meat, all beef bones and beef meat, or beef and veal bone and beef and veal meat, half and half. Garlic cloves may be left whole and later removed by the timid. Barbara uses 4 cloves, cut up, for her family!)

Braise bones and meat in oil until both sides are lightly seared, then add garlic and onion. Sauté for ½ hour. Pour in the celery, carrots, tomatoes and add to the cold stock and water in the soup pot. Bring to a boil, add pepper to taste (celery has salt enough in it), 2 bay leaves (optional), and boil for 2 hours. The meat and soup are a complete meal.

***Pahrtabour* (for eight)**

Dr. Williams earlier listed Barbara's *pahrtabour* soup as one of her prime nutrient choices. Try it. Fall in love with it. It's power-packed. These ingredients, taken as a habit, work wonders in the Caucasus and will for you.

Ingredients: 1 lb. or so of lamb or veal tripe; 2 bay leaves; 3 quarts water; 1 veal bone cut for soup; 2 quarts chicken stock; 2 cups chopped celery; 1 cup chopped onion; ½ cup white cooking wine; ½ cup millet meal; 1 cup chopped leeks; 2 pinches of black pepper and as much salt or Parkelp.

Boil tripe with bay leaves in the water for 1 hour. Discard the water and bay leaves. Cut up tripe for grinding and pass through fine grinder setting.

While tripe is boiling, cook the veal bone in 2 quarts chicken stock for ½ hour, then add the celery, onions and wine. When tripe is ground, add to the cooking soup and simmer for ½ hour longer. Now add millet meal. Cook for 20 minutes more. Add the leeks, pepper and salt (Barbara adds no salt at all), and cook for 10 minutes longer. Serve half. Cool and refrigerate the second half for later use. Keeps one week.

SALADS:

Tarama with Shrimp Salad

Ingredients: 1 tsp. ground white horseradish; ½ cup chili sauce; 1 cup yogurt; 1 tbsp. *tarama* (pink roe); 12 black olives, pitted and chopped fine; 2 tbsp. vegetable oil; 1 lb. cooked shrimp; 4 beds of green lettuce.

Mix the horseradish and chili sauce, yogurt, *tarama,* chopped olives and oil. Add shrimp, stir and portion over lettuce beds. Serve chilled.

Stuffed Artichoke Salad

Ingredients: 4 artichokes (good-sized); enough water to cover; the juice of 1 lemon; 1 clove garlic; ½ cup white wine; 1 tbsp. vegetable oil; 1 hard-boiled egg; 6 pitted green olives; 4 anchovy filets; 6 capers; 1 tbsp. grated onion; 2 tbsp. yogurt; a pinch of paprika; lettuce.

Cook the artichokes in boiling water with the juice of the lemon, half the lemon rind, the garlic, slightly crushed, the white wine and the oil. When an outer leaf comes loose without effort, it is cooked. Figure on 30 minutes or so. (At this point the artichoke may be served as a vegetable if you wish, topped with oil or butter.

To make salad, cool the artichokes and then cut the stem from each. Peel the stems. Press leaves of each down to form four cups. Now remove the chokes, those reddish prickly parts, using the point of a knife, and scoop out the fuzzy innards, being careful not to scoop away any of the meaty parts. The artichokes are now ready to receive stuffing.

To make the stuffing, chop together the egg, olives, anchovy filets, capers and meatier stems, removed earlier. Mix in the grated onion and yogurt. Stir until well blended. Top with paprika. Spoon into artichoke cups. Chill, Serve on lettuce.

Artichoke Filled with *Tarama*
Prepare artichokes for stuffing exactly as shown above.
Ingredients for stuffing: 4 tbsp. *tarama;* 4 tbsp. yogurt; 1 lemon, juiced, in addition to the lemon used above in cooking the artichokes; 2 tbsp. grated onion.

Mix well the meaty artichoke stems, *tarama*, yogurt, lemon juice, grated onion. Fill artichoke centers with mixture. Chill. Serve cold.

***Tarama* Salad**
Ingredients: 1 cup *tarama;* any available roe, cod, carp, halibut, salmon, or sturgeon—whichever is the least expensive; 2 slices large sweet onions; juice of 1 lemon; ½ cup fine whole-wheat bread crumbs; 1 cup vegetable oil; 2 tbsp. fresh parsley; sliced tomatoes; fresh herbs to taste; lettuce or greens as bed. Barbara finds dried parsley flakes or powder tasteless and suspects they are deficient, too.

Blend the *tarama*, onion, lemon juice, crumbs and oil, using about half the oil and saving the rest. When thoroughly blended, slowly add the remaining oil until the mixture has the consistency of sour cream—thick sour cream.

Remove from the blender. When ready to serve on a bed of green lettuce or any green or greens, stir in parsley, mixing with spoon. Add tomato slices and herbal frills to taste.

***Tarama*-Avocado Salad**
A variation on the above.
Ingredients: 1 tbsp. chopped onion, 2 tbsp. *tarama;* ½ cup yogurt; a bed of lettuce; 2 avocados, sliced; 4 hard-boiled eggs; parsley sprigs; chives; pepper; herbs to taste.

Mix the onions, yogurt and *tarama* by hand or blender. Lay out the lettuce bed. Decorate with ½" avocado slices and boiled-egg slices, alternately. Pour the mixture over the eggs and avocados, and garnish with parsley, chives or both. Barbara peppers lightly, and adds herbs (never the same twice). She does not salt.

Cress, Kraut'n'Cottage Salad

Ingredients: 1 cup chopped sauerkraut; 1 pint cottage cheese; a bed of lettuce; a handful of watercress; and a sprinkle of paprika.

Chop the sauerkraut fine, mix it thoroughly with the cottage cheese, spoon the mixture into the center of the lettuce bed, garnish liberally with the watercress and top with paprika. Chill and serve. Barbara is very partial to this tasty salad for balancing luncheons and to accompany full-course dinners.

Fish *Plaki* Vegetable Salad

Ingredients: ½ cup chopped celery; ½ cup chopped carrots; ½ cup chopped parsley; 1 clove garlic; 2 cups water, or water and fish stock—half and half; 1 large whitefish, or any other fish you enjoy cold; 1 lemon; ½ cup chopped tomatoes; and ½ cup vegetable oil.

Cook the celery, carrots, parsley and garlic *al dente* in water, substituting fish stock for half the water if available. Find a use for the vegetable water/stock. (It can be chilled as a drink.) Place the fish in a Pyrex baking dish. Arrange the cooked vegetables around it. Squeeze the lemon juice over the fish. Top with chopped tomatoes and oil. Bake in a preheated 350°F. oven for 1 hour. May be served hot out of the oven as an excellent dinner. As a salad, portion the fish and decoratively arrange all ingredients on lettuce when chilled. In warm weather, refrigerate and serve "piping" cold.

String Bean Salad

A West Point Farms treat that can be prepared any time, refrigerated and used with lunch, dinner, or between meals as a snack, it's delicious.

Ingredients: 1 lb. string beans; 1 clove garlic; 1 small finely sliced onion; 1 tbsp. apple-cider vinegar; 2 tbsp. vegetable oil; pinches of salt and pepper; lettuce; fresh herbs (optional).

Prepare the string beans, trimming them French or julienne, as you prefer. Steam them with the garlic, slightly crushed, whole clove or minced, as you prefer. Steam until *al dente,* avoiding overcooking. Add the onion, vinegar and oil. When cool, salt and pepper to taste. The salad may be mixed with other greens, served as side dish, on lettuce or without, adding herbs of choice if desired. This is a fine snack or summer salad—serve it with dinner, lunch or for munching on instead of sweets.

Favorite Cheese Salad

This salad is so named because you select your own hard cheese to grate. The whole world provides cheeses. Barbara likes unsliced Swiss with this salad, but you may use parmesan, cheddar or a mixture of several hard cheeses, as you like it.

Ingredients: ½ lb. grated hard cheese; 4 hard-boiled eggs, mashed or grated; 1 cup yogurt; 1 tbsp. grated white horseradish; ½ tsp. cumin; a mix of the greenest greens available, including romaine, chicory, escarole, spinach, early dandelion, roccola, or whatever you can combine raw, proportioned as you prefer, experimenting with fresh herbs you learn to like, for variety.

Mix the grated cheese and eggs well, then fold in the yogurt, horseradish, cumin. When well-integrated, spoon into a bowl with the greens, toss, add herbs, salt and pepper to taste and serve cold.

Feta'n'Herb Salad

A natural-goodness cocktail, varied ad lib as an herbal sampler.
Ingredients: 1 cup vegetable oil; purée of 1 lemon; ½ cup crumbled feta cheese; 2 cups finely sliced onions (Barbara's choices are red or Bermudas); ½ cup dill; 1 tsp. chopped basil and/or pinches of chives, parsley, chicory, dandelion, and other available fresh herbs in small but increasing quantities as you try them out—increase the use of those you like and go easy on those you like less. (Hints for other herbs to try are in Chapters 4 and 5, where the nutrient values of so many are given.)

Combine the vegetable oil with the lemon purée, stir in the feta cheese, and pour this mixture over the onions. Garnish by sprinkling in dill. Experiment by adding the suggested herbs to the greens bed and adding them to the mix. There can be dozens of variations, all "dill-licious" and nutritious. If the taste of feta is problematically strange, try other cheeses with it and gradually build your taste for this fine cheese.

Cottage Cheese Melon Salad

A good-sized melon or cantaloupe provides a four-serving-sized seasonal housing for this high-protein treat. Watermelon balls are equally palatable, but without the housing unless you are planning to serve a crowd. By adding other seasonal fresh fruits in a ring around the serving, you can easily build this into a main course.
Ingredients: 1 melon; 1 lb. cottage cheese; 1 cup crushed pineapple, either fresh or canned in its own unsweetened juice, *not* in thick syrup; ½ cup chopped pecans, or other nuts from the shell; 3 small pieces of crystallized ginger, chopped fine; lettuce and/or greens. (Optional as dressing: ½ cup yogurt as topping for each portion.)

Open an end of the melon enough to scoop out its seeds and rindy innards. Peel the melon. Mix the cheese, pineapple, nuts and ginger. Fill the melon with the mix. Refrigerate for 2 to 3 hours. Slice into four equal portions. Serve, surrounded by lettuce and/or greens.

Chicken and Walnut Salad

If you know your way around ethnic groceries (it's never too late to start), keep asking for green nuts and such items as *petmez* and others we mention until you get them. At your stores and health-food shops, talk up the scarce items. Persuade your friends to ask for them, too. Get demand started. Be patient. Persist. Insist. When the stores get the feeling you are a market, they'll come through if they are good businessfolks.

I bring that up because this recipe properly calls for green nuts or green walnuts. The young, not quite ripe walnut has nutritional qualities, as Dr. Williams has mentioned, which are not available in the mature walnuts. Substitute green nuts if you are able. Until then. . . .

Ingredients: 2 cups cooked, diced chicken (this is a great way to consume some of the chicken you used in making stock); 1 cup chopped celery; ½ cup walnuts, pieced but not chopped fine; 2 tbsp. chopped spinach; 3 finely sliced anchovies; ½ cup chopped watercress; 1 tbsp. capers; 1 small chopped onion; 1 cup yogurt; 1 tbsp. vegetable oil; 2 tbsp. apple-cider vinegar.

Mix the chicken, celery and walnuts. Mix all other ingredients well until the yogurt in the mix is greenish. Portion out the chicken on the lettuce. Pour the yogurt dressing on each portion. Serve cold. Decidedly delicious!

VEGETABLES

Spinach and Spinach with Pomegranate

Cultivate the vegetable habit. There is so much good in fresh vegetables, sautéed *al dente* in oil or slightly undercooked, that their proper preparation is worth all your trouble to get them right.

Ingredients for spinach alone: 1 cup milk; 2 lbs. fresh spinach, cold water rinsed if sandy; 1 clove garlic; 1 medium chopped onion; 2 tbsp. vegetable oil, 2 tbsp. butter; 1 tbsp. whole-wheat flour; ¼ cup yogurt; ¼ cup chicken stock; 1 to 2 sprinkles nutmeg; salt and pepper to taste.

Warm the milk. Add the spinach with the garlic clove. Simmer for ten minutes, or until tender. Sauté the onion in oil and butter, add flour, and stir a few minutes until golden. Remove the spinach from the milk, drain and chop fine. Add the yogurt and stock to the onion sauté. Stir to prevent yogurt curdling. Add the chopped spinach, sprinkle on nutmeg, then salt and pepper to taste. Simmer for 5 minutes. Serve immediately. (Use leftover milk in a soup.)

Ingredients for spinach with pomegranate: 1 medium onion; 1 tbsp. oil, 2 tbsp. butter; 1 lb. spinach; a pinch of salt; ½ cup brown rice; 3 tbsp. pomegranate syrup from an Armenian, Greek, Syrian or Near East grocery; and a pinch of pepper.

Sauté the onion in oil and butter until golden brown. Chop the spinach fine and add to the onion. Slightly salt and cook brown rice in the water until water is absorbed. Add the brown rice to the spinach and stir until mixed. Add the pomegranate syrup. Cover. Simmer for 10 minutes. Pepper lightly. Serve hot.

Carrots West Point Farms

Ingredients: 4 medium carrots; ½ cup milk; 1 tbsp. oil; 1 tbsp. butter; 1 tsp. whole-wheat flour; 1 tbsp. chopped parsley; and salt to taste.

Lightly scrape the carrots, halve lengthwise, then further reduce into long slices about ⅛″ or so around. Warm the milk and then add carrots. Simmer for 10 minutes. Heat the oil and butter, and add the flour and parsley. The milk should be mostly absorbed by now in simmering. Pour the oil, butter, flour and parsley over the carrots. Simmer for 5 minutes more, salt lightly and serve. Barbara adds peas only when available fresh-grown and tender.

Savoy Cabbage

This recipe applies equally to regular cabbage.

Ingredients: 1 cup milk; 1 tsp. caraway seeds; 2 lbs. cabbage chopped quite fine; 2 tbsp. vegetable oil; 1 tbsp. butter; 1 medium onion chopped fine; 1 tbsp. whole-wheat flour; ¼ cup yogurt; and ¼ cup chicken stock.

Heat the milk. Put in the caraway seeds, and then add the cabbage. If new cabbage, bring to a boil, cover, turn off the fire and set aside. If not, cook for 5 minutes before covering, then turn off the flame. To make the sauce, warm the oil and butter, add the chopped onions, sauté for 3 minutes, add flour and sauté for 2 minutes more. Mix the yogurt and stock and add to sauté. Strain and add the cabbage to the sauce. Serve immediately. If the cabbage is kept a while before serving, warm again in milk before serving, strain, add to the sauce and serve. (Use the milk in a soup or simply chill and drink.)

Summer Squash

Wash but do not peel your summer squash. The skin becomes tender when cooked and is nutritious and good roughage.

Ingredients: 2 summer squash, each slant-cut into 6 to 8 slices; 2 tbsp. vegetable oil; 2 tbsp. whole milk; 1 tsp. *petmez;* 1 tsp. *origan* (marjoram). Cook squash in all the other ingredients for 10 minutes, or until tender through skin. Learn the least amount of cooking that pleases your family and eat it that way. You should need no other seasoning.

Squash with Yogurt

Ingredients: 1 chopped medium-sized onion; 3 tbsp. vegetable oil, 4 summer squash or 2 butternut squash, peeled and sliced; 1 grated garlic clove; 1 tsp. turmeric; ½ cup chicken stock; 2 cups yogurt; and 1 tsp. basil.

Sauté the onion in the vegetable oil until golden. Add the squash. Stirring, add the garlic, turmeric, stock, yogurt, basil. Lower the heat. Simmer until tender. Serve.

Squash with Lentils

Ingredients: 1 cup lentils; 1 onion; 2 tbsp. vegetable oil; 1 butternut squash or 2 summer squash; 1 tbsp. lemon juice; and 2 cups water.

Sauté the onion in the vegetable oil until tender, golden. Add lentils and water. Simmer until tender (about 25 minutes). Peel and slice the squash, then add to the lentils. Cover. Simmer for about 20 minutes. Add the lemon juice. Stir well. Serve.

Cooked Cucumber

After selecting a young cucumber the same approximate size as the summer squash, peel it lightly or partially and prepare exactly as summer squash, using the same ingredients and the same quantities of each.

Stuffed Cucumber

Ingredients: 2 medium-sized cucumbers, halved; 2 tbsp. red lentils; 2 tbsp. vegetable oil; 1 cup chicken stock; 1 small chopped onion; 1 tsp. chopped parsley; 1 clove garlic chopped fine; salt and pepper to taste.

Peel the cucumber halves. Mix all ingredients except the stock. Scoop out a deep hollow in each cucumber half. Add scoopings to the other ingredients. When well-mixed with the rest, stuff the cucumber with the mix. Place 4 halves in a pan, pour stock over them, cover tightly and cook or bake for 30 minutes at 350°F. Serve.

Eggplant Parmigiano

The "male" eggplant is superior to the "female." It is important to recognize and use only the male. Where the stalk has been plucked from the vegetable, the indentation at that point is round and small on the male and larger and oval on the female. If the stalk is not

removed, you can still tell the male. It's lighter, size for size, than the female. That's because the female has more seeds, which make her bitter as well as heavier. A male about 1 lb. serves four.
Ingredients: One 1-lb. eggplant; 4 tbsp. vegetable oil, ½ cup tomato sauce; 1 large tomato, sliced; and ¼ lb. muenster cheese (Barbara uses muenster, but others may prefer the real thing or a mixture they learn to enjoy.)

Peel the eggplant, leaving some of the skin on just here and there. Slice the eggplant top to bottom rather than across. Put pieces in a pan with the oil. Place the pan under the broiler until the eggplant pieces are golden brown and soft. Remove. Drain off any oil residue. Transfer the eggplant to a casserole, cover with tomato sauce and top with tomato slices. Grate or slice on cheese to cover. Brown under the broiler. Serve.

Okra
Ingredients: 1 lb. small tender okra; ¼ lemon; 1 large onion; 2 tbsp. vegetable oil, ½ lb. small tomatoes, cut up into small pieces; 1 cup stock.

Wash the okra, removing its stems carefully to avoid cutting them open and letting any juice run out. Rub each okra with the lemon quarter. Cut up the onion and sauté in vegetable oil until light brown. Add the okra. Squeeze in remaining lemon juice and add remaining ingredients. Cook over a slow fire until the okra is tender to the fork. Serve.

Eggplant, Okra-Style
Directions for preparing it the easy way: 1 male eggplant, peeled and diced; all other ingredients same as for okra recipe above except the lemon. Cut up the onion. Sauté in vegetable oil until light brown. Omitting the lemon, add all the other ingredients. Cook over a slow fire until tender. Serve.

Artichokes
We had two artichoke recipes in the salad section. Here's another.
Ingredients: 4 artichokes; 1 halved lemon; 1 cup chicken stock; ½ cup vegetable oil; 1 cup water; 8 small onions; 1 tbsp. dill; and ½ tsp. white pepper.

Cut away the tough outside leaves and clean the artichokes well before cutting each in half lengthwise. Scoop out the reddish prickly centers with the point of a knife, and remove also the fuzzy inedible portion of the center, being careful not to take out any of the meaty part. Peel the skin from the artichoke stem.

Rub each artichoke half with lemon, squeezing juice into

each in the process. Place artichoke halves in an enamel pan with the cut side up. Add stock, oil and water, and throw in the remaining lemon parts, too. Put one onion, peeled, in the hollowed center of each artichoke half. Sprinkle dill and white pepper on each. Cover. Cook over a medium fire for 45 minutes. Serve.

Jerusalem Artichokes

If you are not familiar with this vegetable, ask your greengrocer. It is quite different from the ordinary artichoke, and is actually quite another vegetable, having something of the appearance of ginger root. (Grated raw with apple and blended with yogurt, Jerusalem artichoke makes a delicious salad.) Jerusalem artichoke is fruitier in consistency than potato (and a healthful low-calorie substitute), tasting not unlike the water chestnut.

Ingredients: 1 lb. Jerusalem artichokes; 1 small sliced onion; ⅓ cup oil; ½ cup water; ½ cup stock; 1 tsp. salt; ½ tsp. white pepper; and ½ tsp. dark honey (or *petmez*).

Barbara prefers scraping artichokes to peeling them, but scrape them thoroughly. That done, combine them whole with all other ingredients and cook over a medium fire for 10 to 15 minutes, or until tender to a fork. Well-scraped, they can also be munched raw.

String Beans

Ingredients: 1 lb. string beans; 1 sliced medium onion; 4 tbsp. vegetable oil; 1 sliced clove garlic; pinch of pepper; 1 cup stock; 1 chopped tomato; and ½ tsp. savory (herb).

Trim the stems from the beans. French cut or julienne the beans, as preferred. Sauté sliced onion in oil for 2 to 3 minutes until pink*. Add the string beans, garlic, pepper. Sauté for 3 minutes more. Add the stock and chopped tomato. Cook until tender. Add savory, remove from fire and serve. Or omit tomato and savory. Cook the string beans as shown above. When adding remaining ingredients to sauté, also include 1 tbsp. parsley and 1 tsp. whole-wheat flour. Top with a sprinkle of nutmeg just before removing from the fire and serving.

PILAFS

White-Rice Pilaf

Serve with meat, fish or fowl.

Ingredients: 2 cups water; 2 tbsp. vegetable oil, 1 tbsp. butter; a pinch or so of salt; a sprinkle of pepper; 1 cup long-grain, enriched

**Barely beginning to brown.*

rice; 1 tbsp. pignola nuts; and 1 additional tsp. vegetable oil held out.

Boil water with oil and butter, salt and pepper. Add rice. Cover tightly, simmer until water is absorbed for about 30 minutes or so. Remove cover. Stir a little and replace cover, now leaving rice partially exposed for steam to escape. This prevents rice from sticking together. Lightly brown pignola nuts in the remaining tsp. of vegetable oil. Spoon over rice and mix with fork. Serve. A West Point Farms favorite.

Brown-Rice Pilaf
Use long-grain, par-boiled brown rice and 2½ cups of water. Cooking instructions and all other ingredients are the same as above.

White-Rice Pilaf (2)
Same ingredients, same quantities as above, except for using 1 cup chicken stock and 1 cup water.

Brown-Rice Pilaf (2)
Same ingredients, same quantities as above, except for using 1½ cups chicken stock and 1 cup water.

***Bulgur*-Wheat Pilaf**
Ingredients: 1 medium onion chopped; 2 tbsp. vegetable oil; 2 tbsp. butter; 1 cup large bulgur cracked wheat; a pinch or so of salt; 1½ cups stock; and 1 cup water.

Sauté onion in oil and butter, then add bulgur and salt. Sauté for 2 to 3 minutes longer. Bring mixed stock and water to a boil and add to bulgur. Cover. Simmer until water is absorbed—about 30 minutes or so. Remove cover. Stir with a fork to help steam escape. Cover again, leaving bulgur partly exposed to allow steam to continue escaping, continuing to cook until bulgur is firm. Serve.

FISH AND SHELLFISH

Barbara's Unconquerable Sole
Made exactly right every time under Barbara's watchful eye, this dish has charmed even lukewarm fish fanciers away from meat dishes.
Ingredients: 4 sole filets, 6 to 7 oz. each; 1 tsp. whole-wheat flour; 3 tbsp. grated hard cheese, Swiss or white American; 3 beaten eggs; 1 tsp. chopped parsley; 6 tbsp. vegetable oil; 2 tsp. melted butter; 1 quartered lemon.

Dip filets lightly in flour. Mix grated cheese with 1 tsp. of the flour, eggs and parsley. Beat with a fork until smooth. Dip filets in this batter. Cook in vegetable oil over a low heat for 2 minutes or so, then under the broiler at high heat until golden. Remove fish to warmed plates, brush with butter and serve with lemon quarter.

Sole with Crabmeat Dressing

Ingredients for crabmeat dressing: 2 tbsp. butter; 1 tbsp. wholewheat flour; 1 cup milk; ½ lb. crabmeat; 4 tbsp. sherry. Melt butter in a pan. Add flour and hot milk. Stir well and cook for five minutes. Add crabmeat. Cook for 5 minutes more. Mix in sherry.

Ingredients for sole: 1 celery stalk; 1 small onion; 2 tbsp. butter and 2 tbsp. vegetable oil; ¼ cup yogurt; 1 cup cracker crumbs; ½ cup almonds; a pinch of mace; a pinch of nutmeg, 4 sole filets; ¼ cup white wine.

Chop celery and onion very fine. Sauté in butter and oil for 3 minutes, add yogurt and cracker crumbs. Slice almonds fine and add. Sauté until they are light brown. Stir in mace and nutmeg.

Lay each filet flat and spread crabmeat dressing evenly over each. Roll each filet into a cylinder and fix with a toothpick. Pour any leftover butter and oil into a casserole. Place filets into casserole. Pour white wine over fish. Bake for 10 minutes in 400°F. oven. Turn filets over. Bake for 10 minutes more. Serve.

Crabmeat *Plaki* (Vegetable)

Fish *plaki* was offered earlier as a salad with the suggestion that you might prefer it hot out of the oven instead. This recipe is given as a hot dish with the advice that, cooled, served on lettuce or greens and garnished with fish sauce, it makes a fine salad.

Ingredients: ½ cup chopped carrots; ½ cup chopped celery; 2 tbsp. chopped parsley; 1 garlic clove, sliced fine; 1 cup fish stock; 1 lb. crabmeat pieces; 1 good-sized tomato, chopped; ½ cup oil.

Cook the carrots, celery, parsley and garlic in the fish stock until slightly underdone. Arrange the vegetables around crabmeat in a Pyrex dish. Add the tomato and oil. Bake for 30 minutes in a 350°F. oven. Serve.

Baked Salmon Steak

Ingredients: 2 lbs. fresh salmon in slices about ½" thick; 1 cup sherry; ¼ cup yogurt; ½ cup diced fresh tomatoes or tomato sauce.

Place the salmon in a baking pan. Combine the sherry, tomatoes or tomato sauce and yogurt, and pour the mixture over the salmon. Bake for 20 minutes, or until tender, in a 400°F. oven. Bake through but do not overbake. Serve.

Salmon Pie with *Bulgur*
Ingredients: 1 cup bulgur wheat; enough water to cover; salt and pepper (light); 1 tbsp. butter; ½ tsp. thyme; 2 lbs. boned and skinned salmon; 1 medium onion, chopped; 1 cup fresh mushrooms, chopped; 1 tsp. vegetable oil; ¼ cup minced parsley; 1 tsp. fennel seeds, pounded flat; 2 hard-boiled eggs.

Cook the bulgur wheat in enough water to cover for 30 minutes. Mix salt, pepper, butter and thyme, working into the salmon meat with a fork. Sauté the chopped onion and mushrooms for 5 minutes in the oil, and then add the salmon. Stir mixture until browned. Add the parsley, fennel seeds, bulgur wheat and hard-boiled eggs. Spoon blend and allow to cool.

Salmon Pie Crust
Ingredients: 3 cups whole-wheat flour; 2 eggs; 2 tbsp. vegetable oil; 6 tbsp. yogurt; ½ tsp. paprika; 1 tsp. milk.

Sift the flour into a bowl. Break in the eggs. Add the oil. Cut and blend the mixture with a fork until it is crumbly in consistency, as for ordinary pie crust. Add the yogurt. Mix well. Roll out two crusts, shaped to fit a Pyrex dish 9″ square and 2″ deep. Put one crust in the bottom of the Pyrex dish. Sprinkle paprika on the lower crust. Tamp in the salmon mixture, spreading evenly to fit the pan. Sprinkle the rest of the paprika on top of the salmon and cover with the second crust. Brush the top of the crust with milk. Make small slits in the dough. Bake for about 30 minutes in a 350°F. oven. Serve.

Whitefish
Ingredients: 2 large onions; ½ cup white wine; 1 lb. tomatoes; ½ cup oil; 3 to 4 cloves; 1 lemon; whitefish. (Buy a whitefish that will provide four generous portions.)

Slice the onions and cook on a low heat in the white wine for about 5 minutes. Add the chopped tomatoes, oil and cloves. Cook for 5 minutes longer.

Place the whitefish (cleaned and trimmed whole) in a baking dish. Pour the hot onion and tomato sauce over the fish and bake for 45 minutes in a 350°F. oven. Top with lemon juice. Brown the whitefish under the broiler and serve.

Halibut
Ingredients: 4 halibut steaks about 1″ thick; enough whole-wheat flour to cover each steak lightly; 2 tbsp. oil; 2 tbsp. butter; 1 chopped onion; 1 celery stalk, chopped with leaves; 2 tbsp. chopped parsley;

1 clove of crushed garlic; ½ cup of sherry; ½ lb. tomatoes; 1 tbsp. oregano; juice of ½ lemon.

Flour each halibut steak lightly and sauté, 2 to 3 minutes on each side, in half the oil and butter, mixed. Use the remaining oil and butter mix to sauté separately the onion, celery, parsley, garlic, sherry and tomatoes for 10 minutes. Pour this over the fish, topping with oregano. Bake or broil for 10 minutes longer. Pour the lemon juice over and serve.

Halibut in Garlic Sauce

Ingredients: 4 halibut steaks, as above; enough whole-wheat flour to cover the 4 steaks, as above; 2 tbsp. oil; 4 tbsp. butter; 4 tbsp. chopped parsley; 2 large garlic cloves, finely chopped; ½ cup white wine; ½ lemon in 4 slices.

Sauté the floured halibut in the oil for 2 to 3 minutes on each side. Set aside. Mix the butter, parsley and garlic, and lather over steaks. Broil until browned on both sides. Pour on the wine and enflamme. Serve with a lemon slice on each portion.

Trout

Ingredients: 1½ lbs. of trout, either small individual fish or as you find it fresh for four portions; 4 tbsp. oil; the juice of 1 lemon; 1 tbsp. chopped parsley; 2 chopped scallions.

Broil cleaned and trimmed fish in 3 tbsp. oil after washing and drying. Broil on both sides for a total of 15 to 20 minutes, depending on the size of the fish. For dressing, mix 1 tbsp. oil with chopped parsley, scallions and the juice of the lemon. When fish is done, divide the dressing among portions as a topping. Serve.

Dr. Williams wrote about Lake Sevan trout with pomegranate dressing. Few of us will ever taste Lake Sevan's exquisite trout. Our best (and lowest in calories) comes from our streams. But ocean trout is also palatable and lake trout, where available, is quite fine.

Pomegranate dressing would substitute the equivalent amount of pomegranate juice for the juice of a lemon, replacing the lemon in this recipe. At the same time, the scallions would be omitted. Pomegranate juice should be purchasable in Middle Eastern groceries and markets.

Seafood Soufflés

This recipe is for lobster, but crabmeat, salmon or boned meat of sole, used the same way, are equally delicious and worth trying, too, for healthy meals.

Ingredients: 3 tbsp. oil; 2 tbsp. flour, whole-wheat or unbleached; ½ cup milk; 4 egg yolks; ½ cup yogurt; 2 cups cooked lobster meat, preferably fresh cooked and chopped into small bite-size chunks (if cooking your own, lobster pinks in 2 to 3 minutes in boiling water and is done); 4 egg whites.

Heat oil over a low flame in a saucepan, stirring in the flour, then milk, egg yolk, finally the yogurt—one item at a time. Add the lobster meat. Beat the egg white until stiff and spoon it over the top in a layer. Bake in a soufflé dish that has been set in a pan of water. Bake for 1 hour in a 350°F. oven. Portion. Serve immediately.

Lobster Thermidor

Again, the reader can substitute meat of any hard fish, cod, scrod, swordfish, for instance, or crabmeat or shrimp.

Ingredients: 4 tbsp. oil; 2 tbsp. whole-wheat or unbleached flour; ½ tsp. hot paprika (paprika comes mild, medium or hot; Barbara uses the latter—use the one you prefer); ½ tsp. curry powder; ½ cup chopped mushrooms; ½ cup stock (fish if you have it, otherwise chicken); ½ cup fresh whole milk (or the same amount of cream if there's no weight problem and you really want it rich, but avoid powdered or reconstituted); 2 cups (about 1 lb.) cooked lobster meat; ½ cup grated hard cheese (Swiss, cheddar, Romano, parmisan or any you like).

Heat the oil in a pan over a medium flame. Stir in the flour, paprika, curry and mushrooms. Slowly add the stock and milk. Stir until thick. Now put the lobster in a casserole and pour the thickened sauce over it. Sprinkle grated cheese on the top in a layer. Brown under the broiler and serve immediately. Avoid reheating.

***Midia Dolma* (Stuffed Mussels)**

Mussels are seasonals, best bought only when a fish man you trust recommends them. They are easier to manage when larger in size. Small mussels are not recommended.

First soak mussels in a salt-water solution for 2 hours. Then scrub each with stiff brush or steel wool until thoroughly clean. Open each with the point of a knife. Cut off "hair" growth inside and rinse mussel well in fresh water.

Ingredients: 2 cups chopped onions; ½ cup oil; 1 tbsp. chopped parsley; ½ tsp. allspice; ½ tsp. pepper; ¼ cup currants; ¼ cup pine nuts (*pignolas*); 2 cups of water; ½ cup converted rice.

To prepare the stuffing, sauté onions in the oil until light brown. Add the rice and all other ingredients except mussels, continuing to sauté on a medium fire. Pry each mussel open enough to loosen its joint slightly. Be careful: If you get it too loose, the mussel won't stay closed during baking.

When the stuffing has cooked for 15 minutes or so, stir the

ingredients lightly. Pry up each loosened mussel shell enough to insert 1 tsp. of stuffing in each. Close shells over the stuffing and arrange in a pan in layers. Cover the mussels with a plate small enough to fit under the cover of the pan. Add water to cover the top layer. Now cover the pan and cook on low fire for 1½ hours or bake for the same amount of time in a 350°F. oven. Portion and serve.

MEATS

Lamb-Beef *Dolma* or *Sarma*

In all Barbara's meat recipes, the key word is lean. She mercilessly trims fat away. Do likewise. Any lost taste will be replaced by the other ingredients.

Ingredients: 1 lb. mixed ground lamb and beef; ¼ lb. converted rice; 1 finely chopped onion; 1 tbsp. chopped parsley; ¼ cup chopped fresh tomato; 1 cup chicken stock; salt and pepper to taste.

Mix all solid ingredients thoroughly. Hollow out (to stuff) your choice: eggplant, tomatoes, green peppers, potatoes, zucchini squash, whatever. (If you wrap the ingredients in cabbage or grape leaves, that's not *dolma* but *sarma*.) Whichever vegetable you choose, add its edible scooped-out part to your mix. Then stuff four portions. Do not pack the stuffing tightly or overfill. If using cabbage, soften the leaves by boiling in water for a few minutes and cut away the hard parts when removing from water. Grape leaf instructions to come.

When stuffed or rolled (cabbage and grape leaves), place portions in a pan in the stock. Cover and bake or simmer for 1 hour. Serve.

Combination *Dolma*

Ingredients: 4 green peppers; 4 tomatoes; 2 small squash of choice; 2 long, small eggplants; 2 medium chopped onions; 2 tbsp. parsley; 1 tbsp. basil; 1 lb. ground beef, or ½ lb. each ground lamb and beef, combined; ½ cup converted rice; 1 cup chicken stock.

Scoop out the centers of all vegetables. Now mix thoroughly all vegetable scoopings with the onions, parsley, basil, ground meat and rice. Fill the hollows in each scooped-out vegetable with your mix, not tightly or overfull. Simmer or bake in the stock for 1 hour. Portion so as to provide each diner with a slice of each vegetable with its stuffing.

Vegetable Meat Loaf

Dr. Williams wrote earlier about the Caucasus way of stretching meats. This recipe serves four twice. A small amount of ingenuity can stretch this loaf, Caucasus-style, to serve a dozen with little or no more meat.

Remember, in buying meat the key word is lean. Negotiate with your butcher and be sure to get it lean. One way you may vary this dish is by constituting your 1 lb. of meat entirely with chopped beef, or with more or less equal parts of chopped beef and chopped veal, with one-third each of chopped beef, veal and lamb. Add or substitute pork if you like it. But keep your total meat mix down to 1 lb. That's the challenge.

Ingredients: 2 medium tomatoes, chopped very fine; 2 finely chopped tender celery stalks; ½ medium eggplant, chopped fine; 2 tbsp. parsley, chopped fine; 1 large onion, chopped fine; 1 large garlic clove, peeled and squeezed through a garlic press; ½ tsp. thyme leaves; ½ tsp. pepper; 1 tsp. basil; 1 egg; 2 tbsp. yogurt; 1 tbsp. soy sauce; 1 lb. chopped meat(s); a dab of butter. (Once, add 1 tbsp. chopped dill. If you like it, leave it in. Try other herbs and continue their use if you like them.)

Mix together all chopped vegetables, herbs and seasonings except the soy sauce. Turn over in a bowl until well-integrated. Separately, break the egg into the yogurt and stir this into the soy sauce. When well-mixed, add to the meat mix. Add the vegetables, mix well and shape into a loaf.

Put the loaf into a buttered glass baking dish that has been set into a larger pan of boiling water. As needed, replenish the water if it boils off. Cover the baking dish. Bake for 1 hour at 350°F.

People who don't like eggplant may substitute peas, carrots and/or string beans in an equivalent amount.

Roast Beef Filet West Point Farms

Ingredients: 4 lbs. beef filet with all excess fat trimmed away; 1 jigger brandy; ½ cup oil; 4 medium onions; 2 cloves garlic; 1 cup red wine; 2 tbsp. butter; ¼ tsp. mace; ½ tsp. nutmeg; salt and pepper to taste.

Marinate the beef filet in brandy and oil overnight, keeping it in the refrigerator to prevent spoilage. On the following day, finely chop the onions and garlic and then soak the combination in red wine for 1 hour. Braise the beef, turning often until crisply browned outside, rare, medium or well done, as you prefer it.

Sauté the onions and garlic with the wine in butter, adding seasonings. Slice the beef straight and thin, as for London broil. Serve with its sauce.

Beef and Mushrooms

Beef broth is not used in this recipe because Caucasus-style dining calls for very little of it and because Barbara never uses it. You may substitute below 1 cup of chicken stock with 1 tbsp. of concentrate. Beef bouillon cubes added to chicken stock also make a satisfactory "beef" broth for this recipe. Or you may, if you'd rather, use a beef broth you know. West Point Farms diners get their beef dishes with chicken stock and concentrate and love it that way.

Ingredients: 4 tbsp. oil; 1 clove garlic, finely sliced; 2 small chopped onions, enough to fill 4 tbsp; 1½ lbs. choice beef steak, cut in thin slices; 1½ cups chicken stock; ½ lb. fresh mushrooms sliced, 2 tbsp. arrowroot, 1 tbsp. soy sauce.

Cook the oil and garlic for 1 minute in a pan. Remove the garlic, then add the onion and thin steak slices. Heat on a moderate fire until the meat is cooked as preferred. Add most of the stock and all the mushrooms. Cover the pan. Cook for 10 minutes. Mix arrowroot soy sauce and ½ tbsp. stock into a paste. Mix this into the meat-mushroom sauce and stir constantly until the sauce thickens. It's ready to serve.

Caucasusburger

Caucasusburger is a playing field for the imagination when it comes to additional herbs. Experiment in this recipe. Try small amounts for subtle flavors. Write down what you do and preserve the best results as you try others.

Ingredients: ½ lb. lean lamb, double ground; ½ lb. lean beef, double ground; 1 medium-sized onion, chopped; 2 tbsp. chopped parsley; ½ cup tomato juice; 2 tbsp. yogurt; 1 tbsp. oil.

All ingredients are mixed well together, shaped into patties and broiled.

Roast Veal

Ingredients: 4 to 5 lbs. veal for roasting; 2 lemon halves; 3 cloves garlic; 8 anchovy filets; 2 pinches of nutmeg.

Rub roast with lemon halves, squeezing juice onto it as you rub. Slice the garlic and anchovies into bits. Cut many incisions in the roast, filling them with garlic and anchovy bits. Sprinkle on pinches of nutmeg. Roast for 2 to 3 hours in a 350°F. oven.

Veal Cutlet (Schnitzel)

Barbara uses only milk-fed veal, removing a portion at a time from the bone, pounding thin and flat just before preparing this popular dish to order. Each portion of veal is about 6 oz., raw.

Ingredients: 1 egg; 2 tbsp. grated American or muenster cheese; veal cut and pounded for cutlets; 3 tbsp. whole-wheat flour; ½ cup cracker crumbs; 6 tbsp. oil.

Beat the egg and cheese to a smooth batter. Dip the

pounded cutlets in the flour, then in the egg mix, then in the crumbs. Cook on a low heat in the oil until light golden brown. Finish the cutlets under the broiler, watching to avoid overbroiling and toughening this light delicacy.

Veal Parmigiano

Prepare exactly as above. Before putting under the broiler, spread a layer of Barbara's tomato sauce (see recipe) over the top of each cutlet, then top each with 3 slices of American or muenster cheese. Again, watch the cheese melt and turn golden brown—do not overbroil and toughen. Barbara doesn't use Italian cheese in her recipe. Patrons go wild over her version and call it the best they have ever eaten.

Veal Steaks Jambon

Ingredients: 5 to 6 lb. veal roast; 1 clove garlic; salt and pepper; 1 lb. sliced ham; 1 cup white wine.

Cut veal into portions about 1″ thick. Rub both sides of each with crushed garlic. Salt and pepper top and bottom. Place ¼ lb. of ham slices across each veal steak, fold veal over the ham and fasten with skewers. Pour white wine into a roasting pan. Lay in the veal steaks, still skewered. Oven roast, basting frequently to retain flavor. Bakes in a 350°F. oven in about 45 minutes. Serve.

Lamb Fries

You have a diet recipe for this dish in Chapter 10. But we've made so much of it as the unofficial sex stimulant par excellence of Armenian folklore that you ought to have another, with another reminder that it will take negotiations with a specialty butcher to get this item for you.

Ingredients: Approximately 2 lbs. lamb's testicles, diced small; 3 tbsp. oil; 1 lb. small onions (white are best), quartered; 1 tsp. cumin; ½ tsp. allspice; 1 tbsp. sherry.

Brown the lamb in half the oil. Separately sauté the onions in the rest of the oil. When the onions are golden, add to the meat. Add the seasonings. Continue to cook on a low fire for 30 minutes. Add the wine and serve.

Leg of Lamb

Ingredients: 1 leg of lamb (weight varies from 4 to 7 lbs. or so; buy a size you can use, with leftovers in mind); 1 tbsp. oil; salt and pepper to taste; 6 cloves garlic; 1 pint white wine.

Rub the lamb with the oil. Sprinkle with salt and pepper. Slightly crush unpeeled garlic cloves and put in the bottom of a baking pan. Pour in the wine. Place the lamb on this. Bake for 2 or more hours, depending on weight. Set oven at 350°F. As the lamb bakes, stab it with fork prongs, especially in fatty places, to start the fat flowing out. Baste periodically. When tender, remove from the fire, skim and discard any fat. The remaining sauce is excellent to serve on the lamb, sliced.

Shish Ke Barbara

Ingredients: 1 leg of baby lamb; 1 lemon; 1 cup red wine; ½ cup oil; 1 clove crushed garlic; 1 tsp. basil; 1 tsp. soy sauce; 1 tsp. cumin; ½ tsp. nutmeg; 1 small onion, cut in squares; 1 small green pepper, cut in squares, innards removed.

Remove the lamb from its bones, trimming away any gristle and fat. Dice into 2″ squares. Place the lamb squares in a bowl, add the lemon juice, wine, oil, garlic, basil, soy sauce, cumin and nutmeg. Marinate for 3 to 4 hours in the refrigerator.

Preheat the broiler. Spear the lamb squares on a skewer, alternating the lamb with onions and peppers. Brush with marinate sauce and broil until nicely browned all around. Serve directly from under the flame.

***Kufteh* (Lamb Balls)**

Ingredients: 1 lb. lean lamb, double ground; 1 cup very fine bulgur wheat; 1 medium onion, chopped very fine; 1 tsp. chopped parsley; salt and pepper to taste; drops of water as needed; 3 cups chicken stock.

Mix all solid ingredients as if mixing dough. Knead, adding small amounts of water at a time if the dough thickens too much. Knead for 10 minutes. Dip your hands in cold water and shape 1″ lamb balls from the mix. Bring the stock to a boil. Drop in balls (*kufteh*) a few at a time until all are cooking. Cover. Cook for 20 minutes. *Kufteh* will rise to the top of the stock when cooked. Remove with a slotted spoon. Portion and serve. Baste with some of the stock.

Lamb Quince Stew

Ingredients: 1 lb. lamb, cut for stewing; 1 tbsp. oil; 5 small quince; 1 tbsp. *petmez* (or slightly more honey).

Braise the meat in the oil. Slice the quince in strips and core; do not peel. Soak the quince in water until it is ready to cook. When the meat is brown, add the quince and *petmez* (or honey), and cook until the quince is tender to the fork. Very enjoyable. To stretch, add your favorite vegetables. Once you have tried quince, you'll keep it in your mixes.

Pork Roast

Ingredients: Approximately 3 lbs. roast cut of pork; ½ lemon; 5 apple slices; 5 to 6 prunes, pitted and halved; a pinch or so of salt; 1 cup stock.

Rub the roast with the lemon. Make slits in the roast and alternately insert the apple slices and halves of pitted prunes. Set the roast in a pan, salt and pour in half the stock. Allowing ½ hour for each lb., bake in a 350°F. oven. Baste from time to time. Add the remainder of the stock as needed to keep the meat from drying out. Slice and serve.

Pork Chops Caucasus

Ingredients: 8 pork chops; ½ tsp. oil; ¼ cup *petmez* (or ⅓ cup honey); 2 cups whole cranberries; ½ tsp. cloves; a pinch or so of salt.

Brown the chops in a lightly greased pan. Pour *petmez* (or honey) over the cranberries. Add the cloves. Put half the cranberry mix into a casserole. Set chops, lightly salted, on the cranberry bed. Cover the chops with the rest of the cranberry mix. Bake for 1 hour in a 350°F. oven. Serve.

Liver

Ingredients: 2 lbs. beef or calves liver; ¼ tsp. paprika; 1 tbsp. whole-wheat flour; 6 tbsp. oil; ½ sliced Spanish onion; 6 apple slices, ¼" thick; 1 tbsp. honey (or a scant tbsp. *petmez*).

Rinse and drain the liver. Cut into four portions. (Yes, you're better off buying it uncut and doing it yourself just before preparing. Preserves better, keeps its values better.) Season the liver with paprika and sprinkle lightly with flour. Brown over a low fire in 2 tbsp. oil. In another pan, sauté the Spanish onion in 2 tbsp. oil. When the onion is browned, spoon over the liver. Separately sauté the apple slices in 2 tbsp. oil. Dot with honey or *petmez*. When the apple slices are tender, serve the liver over them and garnish with the sautéed onions.

With three separate operations to concern you, take great care to avoid overcooking and toughening the liver. Food values are preserved and taste far better when liver is cooked just enough, somewhat rare. Timing is everything in this dish. Dr. Williams pointed out the worth of liver. Every cook should master its preparation.

Kidneys

Here's another high-value food people should learn to enjoy.

Ingredients: Approximately 1 lb. veal or lamb kidneys (preferred to others, but you should try them all for your own preference); ¼ cup vegetable oil; 1 jigger brandy; 1 jigger sherry; ½ cup sliced mushrooms; ½ tsp. horseradish; 1 cup half'n'half (light) cream (dieters must modify to milk).

Slice the kidneys in small pieces. Heat the oil in a pan and brown the kidneys. When they lose their raw, red color, enflamme with brandy. When the flame dies out, pour sherry over the kidneys, add mushrooms, horseradish and cream. Cook for 10 minutes and serve.

Sweetbreads

Ingredients: 2 sweetbreads; 2 tsp. salt; 3 tsp. apple-cider vinegar; 3 tbsp. oil; 2 egg whites; ½ cup finely ground walnuts.

Soak the sweetbreads in cold water, ½ tsp. salt and 1 tsp. vinegar. Pour off water after 30 minutes. Repeat this process—that is, soak for 30 minutes longer in water with ½ tsp. salt and 1 tsp. vinegar. Drain. Repeat once more and drain.

After the sweetbreads have been soaked and drained for the third time, place them in a saucepan with enough water to cover. Add ½ tsp. salt. Bring the water to a boil, drain and put the sweetbreads in cold water to rinse. Drain off water thoroughly and set the sweetbreads on a paper towel.

Put oil in a skillet. Dip the sweetbreads in unbeaten egg whites, then roll them in ground walnuts. Sauté the sweetbreads until light brown on both sides. Remove from the heat, portion and serve.

Eggplant Omelette

This is a fine change of pace luncheon or dinner dish.

Ingredients: 1 medium-sized eggplant; ½ lb. lean ground beef; 1 small onion, chopped; 3 tbsp. oil; parsley and sunflower seeds, about equal amounts totalling 2 tbsp.; 3 eggs; salt and pepper to taste.

Peel and grate the eggplant. Brown the meat with the onion in 1 tbsp. oil and add the eggplant. Add the parsley, sunflower seeds and 1 egg, and mix well. Heat the rest of the oil in a pan. Beat 2 more eggs, season with salt and pepper, add to the mix and cook in the oil. Turn and cook underside. Both sides should be browned. Portion and serve.

***Soudjuk* (Armenian Sausage)**

Dr. Williams mentioned *soudjuk* and *basterma.* To try *basterma,* buy it in an ethnic grocery. Home preparation of this sausage is hopelessly complicated for the uninitiated. Recipes vary around the world. They vary for *soudjuk*, too, but Barbara's is not too complicated for the venturesome.

Ingredients for *soudjuk:* 5 lbs. ground lean beef; 1 cup very finely chopped green pepper, ground together with the meat; 2 tbsp. cumin; 1 tbsp. paprika; 1 tsp. black pepper; 1 tsp. allspice; 1 tsp. cinnamon. (For sausage casings to hold the mix, order by the pound from your butcher, freezing leftovers for future need.)

Mix all ingredients thoroughly. Refrigerate overnight and mix well again. Stuff sausage-casing lengths with the mix, twisting, but not breaking the casing, every 5" or so. This divides your portions automatically into *soudjuks* (sausages). Punch one small needle hole at each twist—at the top and bottom of each *soudjuk*—to let air bubbles out. Hang entire length of *soudjuks* by an open window in a dry place. Permit to dry out for two weeks.

Soudjuks may be sliced and eaten raw as appetizers, diced into soups, cooked with eggs, sliced as bacon or ham, munched as a snack, added to salads with hard cheese slices or chunks (as a chef's salad variant), used and enjoyed any number of ways, once the family gets the hang and savor of *soudjuk*.

Herissah

The dish of legend, whose story Dr. Williams repeated for you, has undergone many a change and adaptation since it was accidentally created and named. Here is one *herissah,* emphasizing nutrition.

Ingredients: 1 cup polished wheat, bran cover removed (or 1 cup brown rice); 1 quart boiling water; 4 cups shredded chicken or turkey (purists use white meat, others use dark or a mix); 1 pint chicken stock; salt and pepper to taste; ⅛ lb. butter; ½ tsp. paprika; a few sprinkles of cumin.

Put wheat or rice in the boiling water, remove from the heat and soak overnight. Next day, add fowl to the chicken stock, plus 1 pint of the water in which the wheat or rice soaked, and all of the soaked wheat or rice. Be sure that half the boiled water in which the wheat or rice soaked is discarded to get the right consistency. Cook this mixture slowly on a moderate fire until the wheat is softened and the liquid is absorbed into it. As it cooks, add salt and pepper and beat with a wooden spoon until the mixture is smooth and just slightly mushy.

When serving, melt butter with paprika, pouring separately over each portion served. Sprinkle each portion with cumin.

Vegetarian Grape Leaf *Sarma*

Grape leaves can be bought in 16-oz. jars or occasionally can be found fresh in ethnic groceries. Put the leaves from the jar in boiling water for 5 minutes, then rinse to remove salt. Fresh grape leaves are handled the same way but don't need rinsing. Leftover leaves can be refrigerated or frozen until used.

Mediterranean countries all have their own versions of this dish. Here's Barbara's—healthful, zestful, tasty:
Ingredients: 1 cup converted rice; 4 cups chopped onion; ½ cup oil; ½ cup chopped parsley; ¼ cup chopped dill; the juice of 1 lemon; ¼ cup currants; ¼ cup pine nuts (*pignolas*); salt and pepper to taste; two or three grape leaves for each *sarma* to be made; enough water to cover.

Combine all ingredients except the grape leaves and water. Mix well. Cut all stems or pieces of stems from the leaves, which you'll find are small. Place the fibery side of the leaves up, the shiny side down. The stem side of the leaves is laid toward the cook. Spoon 1 generous tsp. of the mixed ingredients on two or three leaves. Fold in the sides and roll up like a cigar. Place *sarmas* side by side in a pan. As they accumulate, they may be piled up to three layers deep. An inverted plate is placed on top of them to hold them in position. Add enough water to cover. Cook on a low fire or bake in a 350°F. oven. Takes about an hour either way. Portion and serve.

Baked Eggs'n'Squash Vegetarian
Ingredients: 2 medium-sized squash (summer or other), grated; 1 cup hard cheese (your choice), grated; 4 eggs, beaten; ½ cup chopped parsley; ½ cup oil, or oil and butter combined; salt and pepper to taste.

Combine all ingredients, mix well and pour into a Pyrex dish. Bake for ½ hour in a 350°F. oven. Caucasus peoples vary this fine meatless dish by adding other vegetables, substituting cheeses, combining cheeses, varying the herbs. It's possible to put together an entire week of dinners based on variations of this dish with no two enough alike to give rise to the accusation of repetition.

A healthful way to vary these dishes is by adding bran, whole grains and soybeans in small amounts for extra nutrition and variety. Toward that end, Barbara wants you to know how to prepare soybeans for serving as is or in mixes like the above.

Soybeans (Soya)
Ingredients: 1 lb. soybeans; 2 medium-sized onions, chopped; ½ cup oil; 1 tsp. *petmez,* or a little more honey; ½ cup tomato sauce.

Cook the soybeans until tender in enough water to cover; then drain. Sauté the onions in a little oil until tender. Add the soybeans, *petmez* (or honey) and tomato sauce. Cook on a low fire for 15 minutes. Serve hot or cold as is, or use soya any number of ways, for instance, as suggested in the recipe above.

Happily, more and more Americans are finding soya, finding it tasty, nutlike when cooked to the right consistency, and a highly nutritious source of protein. If you haven't discovered soya, remember how it turned up in our nutrient chapters and turn to it as a meatless protein source.

BREADS

Multi-Grain Bread #1

Ingredients: 2 packages dry yeast powder, ¼ oz. each; 2 tbsp. *petmez* (or a little more honey); 1 tsp. salt; 2½ cups of somewhat more than lukewarm water; 3 cups whole-wheat flour; 1 cup oat flour; 1 cup millet flour; ½ cup soy flour; ¼ cup rice polish; ½ cup barley flour; ½ cup corn flour; 2 tbsp. vegetable oil.

Mix yeast in a bowl with the *petmez* (or honey), salt and warm water. Holding out ½ cup whole-wheat flour, combine all remaining flours, sifting into your bowl a cup at a time and mixing well.

Spread some of the remaining whole-wheat flour on a board and remove the dough from the bowl to the board, kneading for 10 minutes and adding more siftings of flour as needed.

Clean your bowl, dry and put a few drops of oil in it, spreading across the bottom and sides. Oil the loaf of dough and set it in the bowl and cover with a faintly damp clean cloth or towel. Set aside in a warm place to rise. When it has doubled in size, punch down and knead for another minute or two. Now divide the dough into three equal parts. Oil or butter three 8 x 4″ pans and set in dough, shaped for loaves. Cover and let the dough rise again in a warm place. Bake for about 1 hour in a 350°F. oven until nicely browned. Remove from oven. Remove loaves from the pans. Allow to stand and dry on a wire rack. Slice a loaf as you need it.

Multi-Grain Bread #2

Ingredients: 2 yeast cakes; ½ cup warm water; 1 cup whole milk; 1 tbsp. *petmez* (or honey); 4 tbsp. oil; 2 tsp. salt; 1 cup oats; 1 cup whole-wheat flour; 1 cup unbleached white flour; 1 cup soy flour; 1 cup buckwheat flour; 1 cup rice flour. (When you get ready to experiment, substitute millet, gluten and/or corn for any of above flours, or reduce the amounts of some of the above to include the same amounts of these as well.)

Dissolve the yeast in warm water. Warm the milk slightly. Add the *petmez* (or honey), oil and salt. Sift all flours into a bowl. Work your liquids into the bowl slowly, mixing until bread-dough consistency is obtained. Let this rise for 2 hours.

Put the dough on a bread board, knead down, divide into

three equal segments, place in lightly oiled bread pans, cover with faintly damp cloths and allow to rise an hour before baking. Brush tops with butter. Bake in a 350°F. oven for 1 hour.

Butterless Health Spread

Here with the breads, let us suggest a simple nutritious spread for bread, crackers, *lavash,* which comes next, or whatever, to keep down butter consumption while you balance off your diet with grains.

Blend equal parts of *tahini* (sesame paste) with *petmez* in whatever quantities you can use without keeping it on hand too long. Refrigerate.

***Lavash* (Flat Bread)**

Ingredients: 1 yeast cake; 2 cups lukewarm water; 1½ lbs. whole-wheat flour; 1½ lbs. unbleached flour; 1 tsp. salt.

Dissolve the yeast in water. Sift the flours and salt together in a bowl. Make a depression in the center of the flour mix. Gradually work in the yeast water until you have stiff dough. Knead well, cover and let it stand for 3 hours. You'll have enough dough for several dozen flat breads. Make them all up as described below. Freeze any unused breads until needed.

For each individual flat bread, pinch off a portion of dough about the size of a golf ball—no larger. Flour your board and roll out one portion at a time to ⅛″ thickness. Preheat your oven to 400°F. Bake the number needed for 4 minutes on a baking sheet. Remove from the oven. Brown *briefly* under the broiler. They're done.

Dr. Williams and Barbara labored long on the Chapter 10 diet menus which nondieters should also read for helpful hints. Many beverages shown there, which can be expanded by nondieters, provide healthful drink ideas useful to everyone. So we'll add no drinks here. However, the notion that nondieters will forever give up desserts is ludicrous. Barbara has included a group here—some are on the West Point Farms menu, others were created to combine taste with the useful function of body sweeping. They are reproduced here with the suggestion that people ought not to make a habit of desserts. These are all preferable to available sugar/white flour concoctions with seductive tastes but which serve no useful nutritive purpose. Try these as a way to escape those.

DESSERTS

Anoushabour

Traditionally made for the Easter holidays in the Caucasus, *anoushabour* is far preferable to most commercial cookies, cakes and the like.

Ingredients: 1 cup whole-grain wheat; 2 quarts water; 1 cup raisins; 1 cup dried apricots; ⅔ cup *petmez* (or ¾ cup honey); 2 tbsp. rose water; 1 to 2 sprinkles of cinnamon; ½ cup sliced almonds.

Soak the wheat overnight in the water. Next day, cook on a low fire for 1½ hours. Wash the raisins and apricots. Cut the apricots into small pieces. Add with the raisins and *petmez* (or honey) to the wheat. Simmer together for 30 minutes. Remove from the fire. Sprinkle on the rose water and cinnamon. Add the almonds, stirring in lightly. Portion and serve.

Sesame Crust Apple Pie

Barbara has tried every kind of crust eliminating white flour and concluded Americans will never accept a substitute. For special occasions then, and recognizing that this *is* a high-calorie proposition (which is why Barbara makes it on demand only for favorite customers):

Ingredients for crust: (one pie) 2 cups flour (¼ whole-wheat, ¾ unbleached white); 4 tbsp. oil; 2 tbsp. butter; ½ cup sesame seeds; 1 tbsp. bran; 1 tbsp. wheat germ; 6 tbsp. cold water.

To make crust dough: Put the 2 cups of flour in a mixing bowl with the oil and butter. Work this mix with your fingers until it is the texture of oatmeal. Mix in the sesame seeds, bran and wheat germ. Add water and finger-blend until it is of dough consistency. Knead into a round ball, place sheets of wax paper above and below this ball and roll out flat to a sheet large enough to provide top and bottom crusts.

Ingredients for filling: 6 medium-sized Baldwin or Northern Spy apples; 1½ tbsp. whole-wheat flour; ½ cup brown sugar; ¼ cup *petmez* (⅓ cup honey); 1 tsp. cinnamon; ½ tsp. nutmeg; 1 tbsp. lemon juice; ½ tsp. salt.

To make filling: Peel, core and cut apples into wedges. Combine in a mixing bowl with the flour, sugar, *petmez,* cinnamon, nutmeg, lemon juice and salt. Mix well. The filling is ready to go into the pie.

Put one crust in the bottom of a pie pan so that the crust hangs out over the sides all around. Spoon the filling into the pan above the bottom crust, spreading evenly. Dot with a little additional butter. Cap the top crust over the mix and press the top and bottom edges tightly together to form a good seal. Brush the top crust with milk. Prick the top crust in several places with a fork. Bake for 20 minutes in a 450°F. oven, reduce heat to 350°F. and bake for 1 hour more. It's done.

Bourma

Thousands upon thousands of these pastries have been served at West Point Farms. It is an excellent, simple dessert, served by Barbara Apisson with a scoop of vanilla ice cream on the side. To make the paper-thin dough sheets, see our cheese *beurek* recipe. For *bourma*, start with twelve 10 x 12″ dough sheets as made in the *beurek* recipe or purchased as *filo*. (*Note:* If using filo, prepare with double thickness as you are instructed to with cheese *beurek*.) Cut your 12″ dough-sheet length in two and trim 2″ off the 10″ dough-sheet length. The 2″ strip is laid right across the sheet you have trimmed. You wind up with twenty-four 6 x 8″ dough sheets.
Ingredients for filling: ½ cup mixed butter and oil; ⅓ cup *petmez* (or ½ cup honey); 1½ lbs. chopped mixed pecans and walnuts; ½ lb. brown or date sugar (the latter preferred); ½ tsp. nutmeg.

Mix the butter, oil and *petmez* (or honey). Use this mix to brush each 6 x 8″ dough sheet. Mix together the nuts, sugar and nutmeg. Spread 2 tbsp. of the nut mix across the 6″ width of the sheet at the end nearest you and roll up the 8″ length like a cigar. As you roll, compress the ends about 1″ at either end, so that you squeeze the final length down to about 4″ when it's rolled up. (If troublesome to roll, a clean 1″ round dowel stick can be rolled inside the sheet with the nut mix and gently eased out one side when the roll is made. The compression to 4″ is then made after rolling up.)

Place each *bourma* side by side in a baking pan. Brush the tops with butter/oil/*petmez*. Bake for 30 minutes in a 350°F. oven, or until pinkish tan. Serve those needed and refrigerate or freeze the rest for later use.

Brannies

Barbara has an excellent recipe for brownies which is not included here. This recipe is her invention for family and friends. Health-minded people prefer and are better off with brannies, whose ingredients help provide an internal sweep-down. Barbara maintains that's a lot to get from a dessert.
Ingredients: 5 eggs; 2 cups date sugar; 1 tsp. vanilla extract; 1 cup

unbleached flour; 1 cup carob powder; ½ cup oil; 3 tbsp. bran; 1 tbsp. wheat germ; 1 cup chopped walnuts or mixed walnuts and pecans.

Beat the eggs, then beat in the date sugar, vanilla, flour, carob powder, oil, bran, wheat germ and nuts. When well-mixed, spread this mixture across a lightly buttered 8"-square baking pan. Bake for 40 minutes in a 350°F. oven. Cut into squares. Cool. Serve.

Compote
Ingredients: 1 lb. pitted prunes; 1 lb. dried sulphur-free apricots; 1 lb. dried sulphur-free peaches; enough boiling water to cover; ⅓ cup *petmez* (or ½ cup dark honey); 2 cinnamon sticks; 1 piece crystallized ginger, chopped; ½ tsp. nutmeg.

Combine the dried fruits in a pot. Cover them with boiling water. Set the fruit aside to soak overnight. When turning on fire in the morning, stir in *petmez* (or honey). Add cinnamon sticks and spices. Allow to simmer for 1 hour. Remove the cinnamon sticks. Cool. Refrigerate for use as a dessert as is or topped by yogurt dessert sauce (below). Also good on lettuce as a refreshing salad.

Yogurt Dessert Dressing
Ingredients: 2 cups yogurt; 2 tsp. chopped lemon rind; 2 tsp. lemon juice; ½ cup *petmez* (or somewhat more honey).

Beat all ingredients together, chill, and use as topping for compote, on sliced bananas, or as you will.

Quince Mince
Ingredients: ½ cup chopped dried apricots; ½ cup chopped prunes; ½ cup chopped peaches; ½ cup pineapple chunks; ½ cup chopped quince; 2 tbsp. oil; ½ cup chopped almonds; ½ cup sherry. Use fresh fruit whenever possible, otherwise dried.

Arrange each fruit in its own layer in a small baking pan. Sprinkle oil and almonds over the top and pour on the sherry wine. Bake for 20 minutes in a 350°F. oven. Serve hot.

***Petmez* Pudding**
Ingredients: 1½ cups fine bulgur; 1 quart grape juice; 1 cup *petmez;* 1 tsp. cinnamon; ½ tsp. allspice; ½ cup chopped nuts.

Wash the bulgur and drain. Add it to the grape juice and bring to a boil in a double boiler. Lower the fire and simmer for 1 hour. Add the *petmez* and mix well. Add spices and nuts. Serve hot or cold.

Mahalebi

An Armenian adaptation or forerunner (who knows?) possibly of a concoction served elsewhere in the Mideast as *mahlab,* based on the mahaleb cherry, which in Europe is dubbed *prunus mahalebus.* Experimenters might find cherries or a cherry conserve provocative and pleasant changes.

Ingredients: 2 cups milk; ½ cup *petmez* or honey; ¼ cup water; ¼ cup arrowroot; 1 tsp. cinnamon.

Combine the milk and *petmez* in a Pyrex saucepan and bring to a boil. Mix the water and arrowroot. Stir slowly into the milk. Cook on a low fire, stirring constantly for 20 minutes—or until bubbles start forming on top. Pour into individual pudding dishes and chill. Sprinkle with cinnamon. Serve.

Brown Rice Pudding

Ingredients: 6 tbsp. brown rice flour; 1 tbsp. arrowroot; ½ cup *petmez* or slightly more honey; 1 quart milk; 1 tsp. vanilla extract (or 1 tsp. *mahlab* extract, if available).

Mix the rice flour, arrowroot and *petmez* thoroughly in 2 cups of milk. Pour the remaining milk in a pan and heat over a slow fire. Slowly stir in the entire mixture, continuing to stir continually as mixture cooks for 30 minutes. Add vanilla or *mahlab* extract. Chill and serve.

Dessert Date Sauce

Ingredients: 1 lb. dates, pitted, chopped; 2 cups peaches, fresh in season; 1 cup chopped walnuts; 2 tbsp. peach juice or water; ½ cup brandy.

Mix chopped fruits and nuts, adding 2 tbsp. of peach juice if available, otherwise a few tablespoons of water. Cover with the brandy. Soak for 2 to 3 hours. Chill and use as a topping for compote, pudding, ice cream or as you will.

Sesame Almond Cookies

Ingredients: 2 cups sliced almonds; 1 cup sesame seeds; 1 cup *petmez* (or 1½ cups dark brown honey); 4 egg whites, well beaten; 1 tsp. vanilla; 4 egg yolks; 1 cup whole-wheat flour.

Combine all ingredients. Mix well. Butter a cookie sheet. Use about 1 tbsp. (can be heaping) of the mix per cookie. Spoon out individual cookies on the cookie sheet. Bake for 30 minutes in a 350°F. oven.

Dr. Williams' Closing Note

I have no doubt that certain individuals will *not* maintain their weight even with the strictest observation of the quantities and careful serving of no more than one quarter of these recipes for four. I have seen many patients whose individual chemical/physical makeups defy stringent dieting. For these patients I say our Chapter 10 meals must be a way of life for periodic weight lowering and maintenance of their best health regimens. I say that with regret and not without personal understanding.

For the rest of us—most of us—weight maintenance should not be a problem on meals composed of the above or variations. I have put forth the proposition that good health, good sex and longer years are not possible without good hard work on our parts. I wish I knew a shortcut for you. I don't. Nor does anyone else.

A well-wishing friend suggested that we title this book *How to Live Longer and Be Healthier by Working Like Hell for It.* I mention it to be certain that my readers do understand that we long ago concluded that there is no easy way in spite of the popular books. I simply say, if they don't work and our way does, people sensible enough to take charge of their futures, to take full responsibility for longer, better lives, will succeed in spite of past failures.

This book is intended to rally such people. As considerably less-advanced peoples in the Caucasus have demonstrated, happier, healthier, longer life would be possible for more of us for many years had we not lost some of our basic good habits to "advances" in civilization.

As I come to the end of this effort, I look forward to several things for you.

I look forward to your enjoying tremendous choice, great

variety in nutritious foods, turning away from fat-loaded hamburgers and frankfurters, from fat-larded steaks and other junk-food habits we have cited.

I look forward to what Soviet gerontologists today speak of seriously—achievement of not 100 years as a measure of age, but 200. With what we know today, improved by what we must learn, I see it as possible, and I would love for America to beat the Soviets to it. But it must be acknowledged that their margin in centenarians has given them a long head start on reaching out toward the milestone of 200.

For now, I look forward to many more of you passing 100 and living those extra years in dignity and health and with extra decades of sexual contentment.

Those of you cleverest at using your bodies and our Chapter 10 and Chapter 11 recipes, at employing vitamin and mineral supplementation (Chapter 5 chart) *and* at experimenting sensibly in herbs and botanicals beginning with what we have printed here—*those* among you will gain the most from these words. And your children will gain even more if your new habits appeal to them and overtake them early in life.

I wish you longer, healthier years and all the rewards that are possible when body and spirit are nourished properly as a way of life. Finally, I most sincerely wish you the full fruits of tomorrow's nutritional advancements to make living even better.

Freeing humankind of our self-induced pollutants, both internally and externally attacking us, is a tall order. It calls for governmental and industry underwriting, and speed in getting started. Eliminating the pollutants of external and internal life that shorten our years, we must better identify and use those natural nutrients that lengthen our life spans.

If I were a young researcher just starting out instead of one facing the end of a not unrewarding interlude of learning, work and service, I should address myself to wiping out uncontrolled biologic threats. It should be possible, for example, to recycle necessary viruses, microorganisms and interior chemical systems in insects, plants and animal life. It should be possible to overcome external interference with the survival of man, his animals and his plant life. An area needing research is phytoplankton, a large source of the earth's oxygen.

Yes, man's number one priority should be to save us from various threats of extinction, those facing us as potential sudden catastrophes and those long-range eroders and wasters of human health, not to mention birth defects, too, which, in sum, presently impede the possibility of making 200 years a common life span.

Those among you with stamina and determination to see life on earth improve must demand nothing less of the world's leaders. To accept less is to accept as inevitable further deterioration of yourselves and your world and eventual surrender to the destruction of life on earth by your own hand.

I do not accept that for you. I hope you are up to the fight for your sake, for your children's and for civilization's. Have 100 healthy, happy years.

Index

Note: Page references to recipes are in **boldface.**